Praise for the author's works

'*Sleep Well* is a wonderfully practical, easy-to-read book that will immediately improve your sleep length and quality. A good night of sleep is so important for all aspects of physical and emotional health and longevity. Fiona has combined her expertise in areas of sleep, hypnotherapy, lifestyle medicine and coaching to deliver a scientifically grounded masterpiece. Each chapter illustrates and explains simple habits to improve your sleep and boost your daily living. This is a great investment for anyone who wants to improve their health and wellbeing.'

Dr Robert Kelly, cardiologist

'I can't believe how much better my sleep is. *The Positive Habit* night-time audio acts like a switch, and I am asleep within minutes. I stay asleep all night and I wake up with energy.'

J.H, *The Positive Habit* reader

'*The Self-Love Habit* hypnotherapy audios have changed my life. I am literally asleep within 10 minutes. I have willed myself to stay awake to the end but can't. I have everyone in my life trying it.'

C.G., *The Self-Love Habit* reader

SLEEP WELL

Fiona Brennan is CEO of The Positive Habit, a clinical hypnotherapist, a two-time best-selling author and an inspirational speaker.

Fiona has a thriving private clinic and hosts bespoke wellness retreats in Ireland and abroad. Her first book, *The Positive Habit*, is a firm favourite for thousands. Fiona is a regular contributor to *Newstalk* and *The Business Post*. Fiona recently graduated in Lifestyle Medicine and Positive Health from the Royal College of Surgeons. She also trained under Eckhart Tolle as a Teacher of Presence. She is on a mission to help as many people as possible to sleep well, release anxiety and feel powerful.

For weekly insights and free meditations please visit thepositivehabit.com and follow Fiona on her active Instagram page @the_positive_habit_.

SLEEP WELL

8 HABITS TO HELP YOU FALL ASLEEP, STAY ASLEEP AND WAKE UP REFRESHED

FIONA BRENNAN

GILL BOOKS

Gill Books
Hume Avenue
Park West
Dublin 12

www.gillbooks.ie

Gill Books is an imprint of M.H. Gill and Co.

© Fiona Brennan 2024

978 07171 9915 0

Design origination by grahamthew.com
Design adaption by Bartek Janczak
Typeset by Typo·glyphix
Printed and Bound in the UK using 100% Renewable Electricity
at CPI Group (UK) Ltd

This book is typeset in Alda OT CEV, 10 on 16 pt.

*The paper used in this book comes from the wood pulp
of sustainably managed forests.*

This book is not intended as a substitute for the medical advice
of a physician. The reader should consult a doctor or mental
health professional if they feel it is necessary.

A CIP catalogue record for this book
is available from the British Library.

5 4 3 2 1

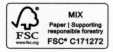

To Aunty Lally and to Olive,
whose breath of kindness soothed me to sleep
and woke me up to a life of safety, joy and love.

FOREWORD

WHEN I WAS ELEVEN, a schoolmate asked me if I'd like to see a picture of a naked woman. This was in County Limerick in the mid-1980s. The most exciting thing you might see would be Farmer Daly driving his hay-filled tractor up the road. Actually, I tell a lie – one day I spied a football sticker of former Manchester United star Gordon Strachan lying under the bars of a cattle grid at the local golf club. That was as exciting as it was frustrating, as his little Scottish head was beyond the reach of my pre-pubescent arms. But, other than that, nothing particularly exciting ever happened in the environs of Ballyclough. So, the prospect of seeing some nudity definitely piqued my interest that day.

I was mildly reluctant to go with this particular chap, as I never quite knew if I was his friend or not. He was my neighbour, was way cooler and tougher than me and had a mind-boggling knowledge of bands with strange names. He was an intimidating sort, and could turn on you at any moment if he felt you were surplus to requirements. But on this occasion I decided it was worth the risk. He explained that the contraband picture was in the adjacent field in an old pumphouse, a building which was basically an empty concrete shed. We set off, and when we arrived he allowed me to enter first because this was my special surprise. On closer inspection of the interior of the damp building, I realised that there was, in fact, no such picture inside and that this was some kind of cunning ruse. Before I knew what was happening, I was flung to the ground and was staring up at his thatch of blond hair and knowing smile. Before punching me in the face, he uttered a sentence that would be so at home in a cheesy movie, it always makes me smile when I think of it. Drawing back his fist, he looked me in the eye and said through gritted teeth, 'You should never fall for women.' And then the lights went out.

Dermot, why in God's name are you telling us this strange, if not a little traumatising, story from your bizarre rural childhood? Well, because this is how our relationship with sleep can be. There are times in our life when sleep seems to switch from being our best friend, our comfort and our saviour to a mysterious entity whom we can't trust, who lulls us into a false sense of security and, just when we need them the most, turns on us like a charismatic bully in a pumphouse. Relationships can only be rewarding when you know where you stand with them, and sleep is no different. We need to be able to rely on sleep, to know that when our head hits the pillow, sleep is our ally and a force for good. Without the right knowledge at our disposal, particularly in times of stress, sleep can drift away from us, and, just like that glorious Panini football sticker under the bars, we can find it tantalisingly out of reach.

The great news is that the knowledge I speak of is between the covers of this book. But this is not just a book; it's a map. A map that will guide you towards not only a lifetime of beautiful, restorative, restful sleep but also those parts of yourself that have been calling for your help and attention. And who better than Fiona to accompany you on this journey? I have sat in her therapy chair, I have interviewed her on my radio show countless times and I have been lucky enough to enjoy her friendship for almost a decade. Her compassion is fathomless, and you will witness this as you turn these special pages. And that compassion will become the golden key to unlocking your sleep journey, because when we are struggling with sleep, we tend to be so hard on ourselves, questioning our abilities, berating our efforts and tormenting those parts of ourselves that are most in need of rest and understanding.

With her unwavering calmness, playful sense of humour and decades of clinical experience, you will get the support and advice you need to change your relationship with sleep for good. Even if sleep is something that you feel is not terribly problematic for you, you will discover new depths to your relationship with it that will reinvigorate your energy, calm your nervous system and boost your lust for life.

I know what it feels like to experience poor sleep. It's draining, exhausting and before long it's all you can think or talk about. It holds us back from living the way we feel we could live and it can create a pervasive anxiety that makes bedtime an unsettling and frustrating experience instead of one of patience, presence and peace.

So, my advice, having been lucky enough to read this book and follow the hypnosis and meditation lessons, is to commit to it. Not because my neighbour will beat you up if you don't but because any relationship needs your full attention. It deserves it and, quite frankly, you deserve it. And when you begin this book and start to listen to these audios, something magical will happen. The doorway of sleep will begin to open up for you and the experience of bedtime will be transformed. I'm not quite able to fully explain it (thankfully Fiona can!), but you will feel lighter, more positive and, of course, your sleep will be deeper and more restorative. Instead of dreading the nights, you will look forward to turning these pages and to the gift of listening to Fiona's voice as it wraps you up in a blanket of deep rest. I know all this because I continue to follow Fiona's course every night. It seems like mysterious alchemy as I drift off each evening and, I have to admit, I feel a little guilty because I get to listen to less and less of the audios, as I seem to fall asleep quicker each time! But I know she doesn't mind; as she will explain, it works whether you're awake or asleep. So, the time for beating yourself up is over. The time for wondering what you've been doing wrong is at an end. This book is the answer you've been looking for.

And, just in case you were worried about little eleven-year-old me, he turned out fine. He never followed that infamous advice that was given to him in the pumphouse that day, and thankfully fell for a very beautiful woman and ended up very happily married. My neighbour and I ended up being great friends and he shared a lot of his extraordinary music knowledge and, more importantly, his record collection with me. One of those records was *Abbey Road* by the Beatles which features the gorgeous song 'Golden Slumber'; it heralds the wonderful gifts awaiting you throughout this book and beyond:

'Golden slumbers fill your eyes,
Smiles await you when you rise ...'

Dermot Whelan, 2024

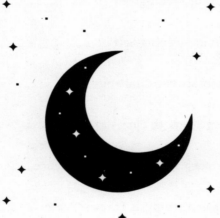

INTRODUCTION

I have slept with a lot of people from all over the world. I have slept with people's husbands, wives, partners, mothers, fathers and even their sisters and brothers. What is most absurd is that I have been given full permission and been invited into their beds. I've slept with people in Australia and America and never experienced any jet lag. To add to this, my husband is not in the least perturbed – in fact, he encourages me to sleep with more people and says he can see the benefit!

Thankfully, the reality is that I am not a nymphomaniac. I am happily monogamous; however, I am a regular bed companion for thousands of people as they drift to sleep – through my hypnotherapy audios.

When I began my career as a clinical hypnotherapist over twelve years ago, I wanted to help as many people as I could. Early on, I began to specialise in anxiety, low mood, burnout and self-esteem issues. I was drawn to these areas because I keenly understand the impact these debilitating states have not only on your sleep but also on your relationships and your sense of self. As I continued to practise and further my training in mindfulness, positive psychology and lifestyle medicine, it became apparent that I had a gift for helping people to get to sleep – and stay asleep. Clients who followed my online courses and read my first two books, *The Positive Habit* and *The Self-Love Habit,* reported their gratitude for finally getting a good solid night's sleep from listening to my hypnotherapy audios; it is no coincidence that the word 'hypno' in Greek means sleep. But I hadn't set out with this direct intention. I wanted (and still want) to help my clients to feel calmer and more positive. As my clients' sleep improved, their levels of stress and anxiety naturally decreased. As they became more mindfully compassionate to themselves and others they began to sleep more deeply. The relationship between sleep and positive mental well-being is reciprocal; each needs the other to thrive.

It became more and more evident that this transition came not by actively trying to help people to sleep but rather by focusing on helping them to feel calmer and more present, so that they were able to fall asleep and stay asleep. I had, unbeknownst to myself, created a successful formula for sleep. I am clear now on what this formula is and why it works, and now it is time to share it with you. As you will discover, this is as much a book about mindfulness and self-compassion as it is about sleep. This is a book that had to be written.

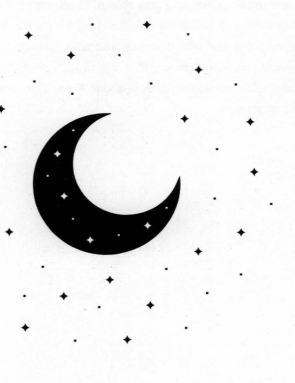

YOUR DECISION TO SLEEP WELL

Oh, the comfort, the inexpressible comfort of feeling safe with a person; having neither to weigh thoughts nor measure words, but to pour them all out ... to keep what is worth keeping, and then, with a breath of kindness, blow the rest away.

GEORGE ELIOT

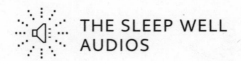

THE SLEEP WELL AUDIOS

All audios are available to download on www.thepositivehabit.com with the password ISLEEPWELL.

Please listen to the short audio track 'Instructions'. It will provide you with an overview of how to listen to your hypnotherapy audios every day.

✦ **Tonight, please start listening to 'Week One: Habit One' of the Sleep Well audios. Please listen to this audio for a minimum of seven nights. Please do not skip ahead to Week Two until you have listened for a full seven days.**

✦ **Please also begin to listen to your morning meditation and your rest ritual tracks each day.**

✦ ✦ ✦

Measure Your Sleep

BEFORE YOU BEGIN Week One of the Sleep Well Programme, please take a moment to rate your sleep. On a scale of 0 to 10, how well have you slept in the last week? (0 is 'terribly' and 10 is 'very well'.) Please use the image on the opposite page to mark where you feel you are on this scale.

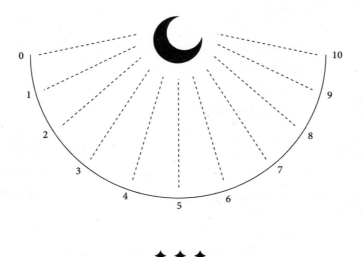

✦ ✦ ✦

One Year from Today

I WOULD LIKE you to imagine yourself one year from now. You catch sight of yourself in a mirror, and every cell in your being lights up. You are glowing, you are full of life and vitality. You feel strong and powerful, you know that you can cope with anything that comes your way. Your eyes sparkle with health, and your entire presence exudes vibrancy. You are smiling at yourself like a person in the first flush of love. You feel present, patient and peaceful. You are brimming with vitality. Your positive energy is contagious, and people are drawn to you. You uplift others and manage to see the positive no matter what challenges you are facing. You are calmer with the people you love. You have more clarity and confidence in your work. You have an abundant supply of love and energy to share. You look years younger and everyone wants to know your secret. One day, a good friend implores you to tell them where your fresh beam of light is coming from, and you succumb with a quiet smile. You want to share it so they can feel as good as you do.

You say, 'I will tell you, on two conditions.'

They hang on your every word. Whatever it is, they want to know. 'Anything,' they say. 'I promise.'

'First of all, you must not doubt me.'

They nod.

'And, second, as soon as you begin to feel as good as I do, don't keep it a secret. Tell everyone you know.'

They nod their heads expectantly.

'I am in a new relationship.'

They never saw this coming. 'With who?' they ask. 'Do I know them?'

'You do!'

This is becoming more intriguing. 'What is their name?' they ask.

'Sleep,' you reply. They seem baffled and even slightly deflated; they had been hoping for something more solid, or even a steamy romance.

It may seem odd to think that you are in a relationship with sleep, but you are. Your relationship with sleep determines all other relationships in your life.

Roles, Responsibilities and Your Relationship with Sleep

THIS BOOK WILL help you, even if you already consider yourself a 'good sleeper' or a 'not bad sleeper'. Wait and see the gold that lies ahead when your sleep has been optimised to its full potential. Whatever your current relationship with sleep is like, I'm honoured you are here, and I value your time. You have many other relationships in your life, and it is hard to find the time to give sleep the attention it demands.

Imagine life is a play and you are an actor. How many roles do you have? Each of the relationships in your life is a role you play, and each one requires you to be fully awake, not asleep. You need the energy from sleep to fulfil these roles. Perhaps you are a daughter, a son, a mother, a father, a romantic partner, a business partner, a colleague, a boss, an employee, a friend, a grandparent, an aunt, an uncle, a niece, a nephew, a cousin, a neighbour, a board member, a community member, a leader, a follower.

Life, however, is not a piece of theatre, even though Shakespeare famously wrote, 'All the world's a stage, and all the men and women merely players.' He meant, I believe, that life is transitory, which is true. But you are not provided with a rehearsal period, nor did you audition for many of the roles you have. Shakespeare went on to say, 'and one man in his time plays many parts'. With this I concur wholeheartedly. Some of these roles you were assigned and others you chose.

Often these roles in the rich tapestry that we call life are nurturing. For example, being a parent or a loving partner is often a joyful experience. However, some of these roles are exhausting and without boundaries. Relationships by their very nature incur responsibilities. But frequently, it is not the nature but the number of roles you are required to play that disrupts the elixir of health – your sleep. In addition, it is often not the roles themselves but the inability to switch off from them that causes you to toss and turn at night. When the lights go out, you are no longer able to distract yourself with busyness. Your underlying anxieties and worries now have your full attention. Concerns about your boss or your family keep you in an unfortunate state of high alert. Each stressful thought is both a threat and a barrier to sleep.

There are many facets to each role. Consider the challenges of maintaining romance while running a house and parenting with a partner. You must change from one role to another within seconds. You are negotiating a work deadline while also trying to organise swimming classes for your child or a hospital appointment for a parent. This transition between roles happens in the blink of an eye and, in the modern era, the touch of a screen.

Dr Matthew Walker, the internationally acclaimed sleep scientist and author of the worldwide bestseller *Why We Sleep*, says, 'Human beings are the only species that deliberately deprive themselves of sleep for no apparent gain. Many people walk through their lives in an underslept state, not realising it.' Often you are not aware of the cognitive and emotional load you are carrying; that is, until you go to bed and your sleep is disrupted. Your mind remains active but your body is exhausted. You are still running through the list of chores for the next day. You are wired but tired.

I am here to help you transform your sleep and, in doing so, transform your life. A well-slept life is a well-lived one.

There is no other relationship in your life that is as important as this one. No other will give you as much and expect as little. Sleep will boost your physical and mental health, help you live longer, laugh more, dampen your fears and elevate your mood. Your relationship with sleep is in direct correlation to the relationship you have with yourself. Certainties in life are few, but rest assured, you are the person with whom you will continue to wake up each morning and go to sleep each night. You are the only person who can improve this relationship. And as in any healthy relationship, trust and relinquishing the need to control are paramount for you to flourish.

Prepare to be in awe of your renewed energy and enthusiasm for life as you fall in love with sleep.

Sleep will soon become a welcome sanctuary, a place of peace to rest in each night. As you drift off every night into a subconscious tranquil bliss, your body and mind will slowly surrender to a profound relaxation that fuels your physical, mental and emotional well-being. The process of sleep allows your muscles to soften, physical and mental tension to dissipate, your heart rate to slow and your breathing to deepen. Sleep is nature's most soothing gift, and your ability to receive it is the greatest expression of self-love.

But you are likely already aware that consistent quality sleep is the foundation for your entire well-being. It's why you are reading this book. However, somewhere along the way, your relationship with sleep has become frustrated and jaded. The joy is gone. You could be feeling desperate and picked this book up as a final attempt to 'fix your sleep'. Or perhaps you've given up battling and moved into a state of acceptance without any hope of reconciliation. It has been like this for years, so it is unlikely to change now. You are resigned to the belief that bad sleep is just part of your DNA. Sleep is elusive, unreliable and unpredictable, and yet as much as you wish you could walk away, you know that you are totally dependent. You can't leave because you need it, so you stay, replacing trust with resignation. You may try to soothe it with medication or alcohol, but nothing seems to make it happy. You're reading this book not out of love, but necessity, which is, after all, the mother of all invention.

When you sleep well, you will release anxiety and feel powerful. The opposite of a vicious circle commences. Let's call it a circle of joy. A core part of my work is to help people to let go of deep-rooted negative thoughts and beliefs that they unconsciously hold about themselves. When you begin to see yourself and the world in a more positive light, you are better able to let go of attempting to control circumstances that are beyond your control.

To go to sleep is to surrender, and to do this on a biological level, your nervous system needs to feel safe.

Do you have a relationship in your life whose 'breath of kindness' soothes your deepest fears? A person who makes you feel safe? Many people seek a feeling of security in other people. It is a mistake to look for this feeling outside yourself. The security you are seeking from other people can only be found within. Once you experience this, everything shifts, including your sleep. Feeling safe is the prerequisite to letting go, and it is fundamental to consistently restorative sleep. Your authentic and most powerful self can only be unveiled to you when your sleep is reliably deep and peaceful.

Neuroscientist, Stanford professor and internationally acclaimed podcast host of *The Huberman Lab* Andrew Huberman says, 'What is not often discussed is how great life is, how much more focused, energetic and how much more positive our mood gets when we are sleeping for the appropriate amount of time at the appropriate depth and when we are doing that regularly. Everything in life gets better when we are sleeping well.'

✦ ✦ ✦

The Seven Main Benefits of Effective Sleep

THERE ARE SO many benefits of effective sleep, and I have listed the main ones below. Before you read them, please close your eyes for a moment, breathe deeply and then bring the snapshot of your well-slept self into this moment.

Open your eyes and imagine feeling these benefits, starting now.

RESTORATION

Your body regenerates cells, tissues and organs as you sleep, providing energy for the next day. You will heal and recover faster from any injuries or illnesses. For example, if you bruise or cut yourself, your skin will heal faster.

MEMORY CONSOLIDATION

Your ability to recall facts and short- and long-term memories is improved. Your ability to focus and communicate your ideas has also increased. You will be able to recall facts and memories and speak with more confidence. For example, you will contribute more effectively in meetings.

LEARNING

Your cognitive function improves and, as a result, you feel more confident. You can solve problems more easily and effectively. What once took you an hour to complete is now done in half that time. You will excel in your studies or at work. For example, you will achieve higher results with less effort.

EMOTIONAL REGULATION

With optimal REM sleep, you feel calmer and more in control. You have transformed chronic stress into positive stress that motivates you to reach your full potential. You respond to situations rather than react to them, and as a result, your relationships are happier. You are emotionally intelligent and resilient. For example, a relationship you find challenging becomes more manageable and fun.

IMMUNE FUNCTION

You get ill less often, as sleep promotes the production of cytokines and immune cells to fight infections and viruses. You have fewer days off and more energy, and you bounce back quickly if you do get ill.

PHYSICAL PERFORMANCE

You have increased fitness levels as sleep improves reaction time, coordination and endurance. You are physically stronger; you can carry heavy bags and walk or run upstairs more easily. You have more physical stamina for day-to-day chores like housework, bending and lifting things.

INCREASED LONGEVITY
You are at a lower risk of developing a life-threatening disease. Sleep reduces inflammation in your body – inflammation is a key contributor to the ageing process. You will live long enough in good health to play with the younger generations in your family and circle of friends.

While researching this book, I read countless books and articles on the most up-to-date sleep science. It is startling how much science has uncovered in the past 20 years about why we sleep. But however educational this science is, it is not always conducive to helping people who suffer from somnophobia, also known as sleep anxiety. This is when the build-up of pressure before going to bed intensifies. A person feels anxious because they can't sleep, and their anxiety prevents them from falling asleep. Too much knowledge can, ironically, create dread around sleep rather than encouraging it. If your system is overstimulated, it simply can't surrender to sleep.

In the early stages of this research, I found myself unintentionally falling victim to this information. I became affected by the volume of sleep science and stressed that should I miss an hour's sleep or break my routine, I'd die early and most certainly with dementia! It was then I knew I had to take a fresh approach based on my success to date in helping people to sleep. This is not another sleep book recounting the negative effects of poor sleep on your brain and body. I am offering you a unique and proven path to wake up to who you are so that you can sleep well night after night.

Rest assured I will provide you with solid sleep science. I have carefully analysed the data to provide you with the ingredients of what makes a person a good sleeper rather than what happens when you don't sleep well. I have unearthed how integral your thoughts and expectations are to your ability to sleep. All will be revealed, and you won't look back.

You may know a person who says, 'I have always been a good sleeper, touch wood.' As if sleep is not a gift given to all of us.[1] When you encounter this 'good sleeper', you may feel an unwelcome spark of envy and a low rise of anxiety in your tummy, as this blessed person describes how they get to sleep quickly and stay asleep all night. Or perhaps you remain apathetic. You have a stale acceptance of your fate and believe that sleeping well is something for other people, not you.

Sleep is not a competition and even for those 'good sleepers' out there, the quality of their sleep can always be tweaked and improved upon. It is, as Andrew Huberman points out, the appropriate amount *and* depth of sleep that elevates a good sleeper into a great one.

You will discover and experience how to change your life while you sleep by reprogramming your subconscious with positive and peaceful suggestions. Night after night and day after day, you will bask in the glory of a well-slept life. If life is a play, then I'm your director, but the only role you have is to relax. Take my faithful hand and let me guide you to sleep each night. Have faith in my kindness, experience and expertise to open the door to sleep, to rekindle trust in yourself.

✦ ✦ ✦

A Story of Transformation: Fionnuala

ON A COLD, bright January day in 2021, I met Fionnuala for the first time. She is a successful professional vocalist and violinist who is a core member of the Celtic-Nordic group Secret Garden, which won the Eurovision Song Contest in 1995. The country was in another lockdown, so rather than meet in my office, we went for a walk in a local park. Fionnuala told me about the challenges in her life, as is common in a first consultation.

As we walked, Fionnuala also informed me how badly she struggled with sleep, which was why she had contacted me. She was clearly exhausted and was suffering from 'sleep anxiety'. Her sleep was very broken, and she had no idea of how many hours a night she was getting, apart from that it was very few. Fionnuala recalled her sleep first becoming disturbed around the age of thirty. She was now in her late fifties. Almost two decades of suffering.

Fionnuala's sleep issues first began in an anxious period of her life and had escalated since then. She was literally afraid of sleep. Bedtime loomed ahead of her each day as a source of dread. She had no faith in her ability to sleep. I listened deeply, and when I spoke, I shared my insight that Fionnuala's sleep issues went far beyond the confines of her bedroom and that her fear of sleep was also a fear of life. I explained that her initial anxiety had found a home in sleep and that for her to sleep again, we needed to remove the urgency from the situation. When you desperately want something, it creates stress, and cortisol rushes through your veins, which makes sleep impossible.

As I spoke, I saw that familiar look in Fionnuala's eyes. I've seen it in many clients over the years. This look is subtle; it is a mix of scepticism, impatience, hope and a deep-down inner knowing that what I say could be true. Often, it's not what they want to hear. Fionnuala, a very intelligent person, understood me on an intellectual level, but she didn't truly believe that if we focused on alleviating her anxiety she would sleep better. When a person is suffering, they just want a solution – and fast. Perhaps you are the same. This is understandable, but this wanting is at the root of what perpetuates the problem.

Your mind is not a switch that you turn on or off. It is a delicate system that dims slowly. Your mind requires regular intervals of rest and relaxation during the day and time at night to slowly glide from wakefulness into sleep.

Fionnuala very kindly agreed to share her story to help you. She will explain in her own words what brought her to my door (or in this case the park) that day. Her story is not perfect, it might not even be ideal, but it does show what is possible.

I got used to the habit of being a bad sleeper. Perhaps it had accumulated over the years. When I was a child, I was told I was the laziest of the five children in my family. People would say it is the opposite now. From a very young age I have had very poor circulation and really felt the cold. My parents had to regularly wake me up during the night if my temperature was too low and try and get my circulation going again. Even with a warm house, my body temperature used to dip very low. Maybe these interruptions could have been the start of my disrupted sleep, as the rest of my family don't have these issues.

Adult life, the everydayness of working, the high stress of the job I do, and juggling too many things made sleep difficult. I used to have very bad nightmares and night terrors. My husband would regularly have to wake me during the night if I began crying in my sleep. I am still not sure why I routinely had bad nightmares and terrors. Maybe it was some unprocessed trauma, as I am a pretty happy and contented person and luckily in a great relationship. But maybe during all the years of my career I have absorbed a lot of stress and it came out in my sleep. Some nights I would feel paralysed and couldn't move my arms or legs. It was terrifying to seem to be awake but not be able to move.

A lot of my recurring nightmares came before a tour. It was probably the subliminal worry of going back on stage and that whole thing of 'Am I good enough?' Sometimes the dreams are about my Leaving Cert, and I'm so many years away from my Leaving Cert now, but in the dream I realise the maths exam is next week and I haven't done a thing. Another one is that I am back in the orchestra (which, again, is so far back in my career) and I can't make it to the stage. We always had to wear all black and I dream that I can't find a piece of clothing, or my violin has gone missing. I never make it to the stage, as I always wake up.

In my thirties I stepped up and out in my career. I left the concert orchestra, I won the Eurovision, I started a new group – Secret Garden – and the pressure was huge when I stepped out of my comfort zone and left a permanent, pensionable job behind.

I was on the road all the time in my mid-thirties, I had a flourishing career, and it was fantastic. But I also had the pressures of being a woman, with a biological clock that was ticking. I started questioning myself and knew with all the traveling the opportunity to settle down and have children was disappearing; that, along with the incredible jet lag from constant flying through many time zones, probably played big time into numerous sleepless nights. Those sleepless nights were a total waste of time, I can see that now. However, it is far better to follow your dreams than to back into a corner out of fear. My sleep could have been better, but I would not have been fully living. I don't regret anything I have done, and yes, it would have been easier with better sleep.

But I pushed myself. I am working with people who do that all the time. I was surrounded by people [who didn't sleep]. I remember my partner in Secret Garden – Rolf Lovland – and me working in LA in Hans Zimmer's studio, which was a great experience. Hans was working on a soundtrack for the *Last Samurai* movie score. He had a big sign in his studio that said, 'Sleep is for wimps.' That was the motto – it's the result that matters, it has to be done.

I remember doing three days and nights without sleep to get a production ready. Work came before sleep. We have more awareness of how to deal with things now, there are more tools. If you are having anxious moments, there are ways of dealing with it. I have changed a lot, but I always need to keep an eye on it.

I am lucky it didn't show on my face. I put on make-up and my game face and off I went. I also made up for it with naps. Now, I go to bed early and I love getting up early, I've always been a morning person, but because of my career, I was forced to become a night one. I functioned without great sleep, and some part of me adapted. But it became a serious issue before a performance, and that is where self-medication began to creep in. I had tried everything, different beds, mattresses, linen, darkness, no TV, no phone, and none of that made any difference.

I tried all the good sleep habits, but nothing really changed until I met Fiona. When I met Fiona, I had just been through breast cancer, and I didn't realise how disruptive it was. I was able to deal with the process and the treatment, but my sleep was so bad. It was the hangover from cancer. In my case, I had been on HRT, and I thought it was fabulous, but I had to abruptly stop taking it once I was diagnosed. When I started the perimenopause–menopause journey, nobody was talking about it. It's part of being a woman in mid-life that you have a sleep issue as we are aware our declining hormones don't do us any favours with sleep and that breeds anxiety, and it becomes a vicious cycle.

I had started to take sleeping pills and Xanax; I had never done that before. Cancer anxiety had shaken me so badly, even though I kept a very good front up. It shook me to the core. I felt like I needed the drugs, but I knew that this was not where I wanted to be long-term. It's not who I am. I am so aware of health in the big picture, that this was not the road I wanted to stay on. I didn't want to be relying on them every night. You start them and it is very hard to stop them.

During the cancer treatment, I would lie down at night and all the feelings I hadn't dealt with in the day would wash over me. The anxiety was so painful, and it seemed to come from nowhere. I was lying in my bed, I was responding well to the treatments, I have a lovely home, I have my husband and our dog. There was nothing threatening me and I felt so grateful for all I had, yet my whole system went into fright mode.

When I met Fiona, I was desperate. I thought, 'Can she fix me? And if so, how quickly?' Through the hypnotherapy audios, I was able to deal with the emotions I wasn't suppressing any more with medicine.

Hypnotherapy is the most useful tool that I have ever come across. It transformed me. I love that hypnosis works so fast and that it works subliminally. I am not a good meditator; I do mindfulness every day but find it hard to quieten the monkey brain. What I love about Fiona's hypnotherapy audios is the fact that I just put them on, and it doesn't matter if I zone in or out, they are working. That really appealed to me. They became my new routine. I still use them. They took away the fear of sleeping.

Now all I need is my phone. I turn on the audio tracks, I turn off the lights, and I am gone. If I am still awake at the end, it doesn't matter. If I fall asleep during it, it doesn't matter. If I don't fall asleep, it is OK. I am not fighting sleep. I'm not afraid of sleep any more.

People who are afraid of it, are fighting it, they are looking at the clock in the middle of the night and thinking, 'Oh Jesus. It's four o'clock, help!' I used to always be terrified of four o'clock in the morning because I heard so many people died at that time. My mom died at 4.07 a.m. I was with her, and this is sort of funny, I was looking at the clock, and I said, 'Mum, please do not go at 4 a.m., you know how I feel about 4 a.m.,' and then she went at seven minutes past, and I thought, 'You must be joking!' Now, if I am awake at that time of night, I just talk to her. I say, 'You are having the last laugh at me.' But it has totally changed how I view that time in the morning. I reframed it. I couldn't have done that without the hypnosis.

I am not using up energy during the night to fight an issue that is designed to help me relax and recover, that battle is gone, and I now have more energy during the day. Things like air travel had become such a pain; if there was a delay or people in the queue were taking forever, in the past those things got to me, and it was exhausting. You are living an exhausting life when you don't have to be.

I just love that the subliminal messages of the audio are feeding the subconscious. It's like doing something at speed. With psychotherapy, you could spend so long trying to get to the same point, whereas with hypnosis it is like 80 per cent quicker, and that really appeals to me. I know that the shift happens quickly but to sustain it I have had to do more work with Fiona, and she has helped me to understand why I react the way I do and not to be afraid of the everydayness of living. I definitely feel I am different from who I was two years ago. I am less anxious and less stressed.

Everything in my life is slightly easier. For instance, I am recording at the moment; in the past I would have rehearsed and rehearsed for hours before I would record even one note. Now, I am much more relaxed and fluid, I am mentally stronger, which also gives a sense of freedom, and the process of recording, which I love, seems to be easier.

The way I play the fiddle has changed. You can't be tense when you play; you have to let everything relax, to let everything flow. If you push or try too hard, you are going to change the sound. I feel I am now producing a stronger and better sound, which is fantastic after such a long career. Sleep is the same. You just have to allow it.

Fionnuala opened her door to sleep, and throughout this eight-week programme you are learning to do the same. You are the host; sleep will come back every night when it feels that your home is a place of peace, a refuge to rest from the external world. The removal of roles, expectations and pressure creates a loving space to rest in.

One of the most important things is to remove the obstacles at your door, so sleep has a clear entrance. One of the main hurdles to sleep, regardless of any challenges you may have right now (perhaps a young baby, menopause or chronic pain), is an overactive mind. When you learn the art of slowing it down, you literally step out of your own way.

You allow nature to do what it does best – to heal you physically, mentally and emotionally.

✦ ✦ ✦

The Law of Least Effort

THE LAW OF Least Effort is based in Eastern philosophy and is Law Number Four in Deepak Chopra's book *The Seven Spiritual Laws of Success*. The principle of this law is that you flow through life in the same way as nature, with effortless ease. Grass does not try to grow, it grows. You don't try to go to sleep, you sleep. I have indirectly been applying the Law of Least Effort to help people to get to sleep, and it has been transformative.

> **It is worth noting that the Law of Least Effort is not the law of *no* effort.**

Sleep is a serious issue that you need to take lightly; in other words, you need to prioritise your sleep without making a fuss. You will learn to allow sleep to come to you by creating a welcoming physical, mental and emotional environment. Setting an intention sends a clear message to your subconscious that you expect and allow sleep to come to you. By gradually implementing the practical habits you will learn each week, you are illustrating the difference between least and no effort. The eight habits also reinforce the intention. Your words are not empty. Positive lifestyle changes require commitment. Now is the time to start afresh: no matter how tumultuous your relationship with sleep has been in the past, you create a blank slate – a new beginning.

✦ ✦ ✦

The Sleep Survey

IN THE NEXT section, I will help you to set a clear intention of why you wish to change your relationship with sleep, and you will also commit to this process with me as your guide. I will clearly outline how to use the book, including listening to your night-time audios. You will then be ready to begin the programme, which acts as a lifelong companion that you can rely on night after night.

Let's start with a practical review of your sleeping habits, including your lifestyle and sleeping environment, and then move on to the psychological and emotional level. You will retake these same surveys at the end of this eight-week programme.

Please note that there is no judgement of the answers you provide. Be honest with yourself – this is a private exercise, and we are not seeking perfection now or at any stage throughout this programme.

Answering these questions will give you an idea of what part of your lifestyle is impacting your sleep and how you can start to make changes that will allow sleep to come easily. Each change you make in your self-care routine is an act of self-love. When you love someone, you care for them.

	Today	At the end of Week Eight
Your sleep habits		
What time do you get up?		
Do you feel groggy or refreshed when you rise?		
Do you get outside into natural light within 30–60 minutes of rising if the sun has already risen?		
Do you use an artificial light therapy lamp in winter when you rise before sunrise?		
Do you meditate in the morning?		
Do you ease yourself gently into the day?		
How soon after waking do you check your phone?		
How much light exposure do you get as the day goes on?		
Do you get outside at sunset?		
Do you have excessive sleepiness during the day?		
Do you rest or relax during the day?		
Do you take a nap?		

Do you experience an afternoon slump?		
Do you reach for sugar in the afternoon?		
Do you reach for caffeine in the afternoon?		
Are you on a screen in the 60 minutes before bed?		
Do you have a bedtime routine to help you unwind, for example, meditation, journaling or reading?		
Do you listen to hypnotherapy audios or guided sleep meditations to help get you to sleep?		
What time do you go to bed?		
How many hours are you in bed?		
How many hours, on average, do you sleep?		
On a 'good' night, how long does it take you to sleep?		
On a 'bad' night, how long does it take you?		
Do you wake up during the night?		
If yes, how many times?		

If yes, how long does it take you to go back to sleep?		
Do you recall your dreams?		
Do you have disturbing dreams/nightmares often?		
Do you have a baby or young children who wake you up?		
Are you caring for another person such as a parent during the night?		
Are you perimenopausal or menopausal?		
Do you have a chronic health condition?		
Are you on medication that interferes with your sleep?		
Have you any specific diagnosis of a genetic sleep disorder?		
When was the last time you had a cold or virus?		
Do you drink alcohol? If so, how much and how often?		
Do you practise yoga or a mind/body exercise routine, such as tai chi, at least once a week?		

Do you dim the lights in your home at least one hour before bed?		
Do you enjoy time alone?		
Do you laugh often?		

Your Sleeping Environment

Do you sleep alone or with a partner?		
Does your partner snore?		
Do you snore?		
Is your bed comfortable?		
How old is your mattress?		
Is your bedroom free of clutter?		
Is the colour and design of your bedroom calming?		
Is the house quiet when you go to bed and during the night?		
Is your room temperature correct for sleep (15 to 19 degrees Celsius)?		

Do you have a pet? If so, do they sleep in your room or disturb you during the night/early in the morning?		
Do you watch TV/Netflix/scroll the internet in bed before sleep and/or at any other time?		
Do you read before you sleep? If so, is the material you read calming?		
Do you study or work in bed?		
Do you smoke prior to bed or if you awaken during the night?		
Do you snack before bed or if you awaken during the night?		

Psychological and Emotional Component

Do you believe you are a good sleeper?		
If not, how old were you when you first started to believe you were a bad one?		
If someone asks you about your sleep, what do you say?		
Do you talk about sleep a lot?		

Do you worry about going to bed and not being able to sleep, or that you will wake early and not be able to get back to sleep?		
Do you believe you are a light sleeper?		
Do you ruminate on your day when you get to bed? For example, do you go over what you said or didn't say, did or didn't do?		
Do you start to plan the next day and recall all the items on your to-do list that you haven't done?		
Do you worry about your future in general?		
Do you worry about a loved one?		
Do you worry about your health last thing at night?		
Do you sometimes have anxiety that you can't explain if you wake up in the middle of the night?		
Do you feel any pain in your chest or heart area as you go to sleep or if you wake up?		
Do you look forward to going to bed?		
Do you feel safe as you go to sleep?		

And finally, answer these.

Issues Impacting Sleep Quality	True	False
I have performed badly at work during the day because of sleepiness.		
I am likely to fall asleep in front of the TV or if I am at the cinema or theatre.		
I am likely to fall asleep if I am a passenger in a car at a time I wouldn't normally feel tired.		
Going to the toilet at night is a problem as I struggle to get back to sleep afterwards.		
I am on medication that could be interfering with my sleep.		
I am on a sleeping tablet and want to come off it.		

✦ ✦ ✦

How Present Are You?

IN WEEK THREE, I talk about the importance of waking up to life so that you can sleep fully, and later on in Week Six: Sleep Strength One – Presence, I ask you to explore your relationship with the present moment.

The mind, when left to its own devices, will stray to the past and to the future, as if this moment now is somehow inadequate, something to be endured until some future, happier moment. This 'better' moment, of course, never comes. As you sleep more deeply, you are in a position to see through this illusion and to feel more clearly the power of presence. In light of this, I would like you to complete one last questionnaire.

Please answer each question as honestly as you can. Don't reflect for too long – just go with the first answer that comes to you.

In the past month have you:

	Today		At the end of Week Eight	
	Yes	No	Yes	No
Found yourself ruminating on the past?				
Found yourself worrying about the future?				
Found your mind overanalysing what someone meant by a comment they made?				
Found it hard to focus your attention on the task at hand?				
Found your 'to-do list' interrupting your peace at night while going to sleep, or during the day if you are relaxing?				
Tuned out of a conversation with a loved one as you get lost in your own thoughts?				
Felt overwhelmed by not having enough time to do all you need/want?				

Felt impatient when something small didn't go your way, e.g. sitting in traffic, losing something or making a small mistake?				
Had invasive thoughts about what people will think of you if you do or say something that you think they won't like?				
Found yourself constantly in planning mode so that you are missing the moment?				

For each 'No' answer, give yourself one mark. The higher the marks out of ten, the higher your level of presence is. Remember that this is not a competition but simply an opportunity to learn about yourself so that you can gradually awaken to presence.

At the end of the eight weeks, make sure to return here and be proud of how much better your relationship with sleep is. Specifically, notice what has changed.

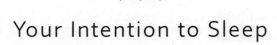

Your Intention to Sleep

RETURN TO THE image of yourself in the mirror, your well-slept self one year from now – unwired, untired. Visualise yourself as clearly as you can, having transformed your stale relationship with sleep into one that is sublime. You love and accept yourself as you are, and any pressure to get to sleep and to stay asleep is in the past. You know how to rest, to relax, to let go, and as a result, you are sleeping well night after night.

Your reflection glows with health and wellness, but I want you to look beyond the physical, and connect to the inner feeling of positive energy flowing through your veins. This is the energy you create, and it is not dependent on garnering approval, pleasing others or accomplishing something. You are quietly confident and have an overpowering desire to help others feel as alive as you do.

As I have mentioned, being a great sleeper does not mean being a perfect one. You will have some nights that are better than others, depending on your particular challenges. However, for your continued progress, you need to make a conscious choice to soak in the benefits, no matter how incremental they are. Remember we are in no rush. You won't feel each one every day; for example, you may feel calmer one day but still struggle to recall the name of a film you watched.

Take a moment and ask yourself, why are you reading this book? Please, go a little deeper than 'I want to improve my sleep.' I need your deeper motivation. Ask yourself how being a good sleeper will change your life. Take time to explore the positive impact that high-quality and consistent sleep will have on your life. Find your specific and subjective reasons for becoming a better sleeper. For example:

✦ 'I will feel like myself again.'

✦ 'I will laugh more.'

✦ 'I will be able to manage stress.'

- 'My relationships will be healthier.'

- 'I will feel energised.'

- 'My appearance will be fresher.'

- 'I will be able to focus at work.'

- 'I will be calmer with my loved ones.'

- 'I will have the confidence to make a change in my career.'

- 'I will be able to recover from my illness.'

- 'I will have the energy I need to spend time with my children.'

- 'I will live longer and be there for my family and/or have the health, vitality and enthusiasm to travel, to create, to continue to contribute to society.'

No doubt it is a combination of all the above, but choose one or two things that resonate and be as specific as you can.

Write your answer below.

I am reading this book because _____

_____

Your answer is your intention, and it is the purpose of our time together.

You need to be devoted to your intention and remain faithful to it, regardless of any challenges or distractions that arise. If you are committed to the process and then your work gets particularly busy or you or a loved one gets ill, for example, your intention to sleep well is not sacrificed. When life becomes more difficult, it's more important to remain steadfast in your intention.

In stressful times, most people sacrifice their sleep and rest time, and they drop their self-care rituals at a time when they need them most.

However, your intention also needs space to be flexible. Choose to rely on the energy of devotion rather than discipline. Care for yourself in the same way you do for a person you love, do your best and forgive yourself when you miss out or mess up. A handy rule to recall is: if you miss one night of listening to your Sleep Well hypnotherapy audios, listen again the next night. Simple.

✦ ✦ ✦

The Sleep Contract

NOW THAT YOU have learned the benefits of effective sleep, can visualise your best-slept self, have a clear understanding of your current sleep habits and, most important, have a highly motivating and personal intention of why you are choosing to sleep well, it is time to truly commit. The best way that I know to make a strong commitment to something important is to sign my name on the dotted line. I also want to make sure that you are fully dedicated to improving your sleep, that you are willing to do your best, which is all any of us can do.

So here it goes: you and I are going to sign a sleep contract. Your relationship with sleep is, after all, the most important relationship in your life.

> *I, Fiona Brennan, am committed to helping you to sleep peacefully to the best of my ability. The tools and insights shared in this book are based on up-to-date science and my wealth of clinical experience.*

Signed Fiona Brennan

> *I, ...,*
> *am committed to following the programme to the best of my ability and devoting myself to the love of sleep. I will be kind to myself if I miss one night of the eight-week programme, and I will simply start again the next night.*

Signed ....

✦ ✦ ✦

The Sleep Well Programme

CHOOSE ONE THING you are accomplished at and feel confident about. This could be playing tennis or a musical instrument, cooking beautiful meals for your family or an aspect of your job that people come to you for help with. What does it feel like to know you can do this activity well? What steps do you use to ensure you continue to do a good job? Perhaps these are not always in the exact same order, and you bring a touch of magic – something new – each time you do it. Still, you have the same set of steps that you follow, and it works. The Sleep Well Programme is the same: you follow the steps to become and remain a good sleeper.

This book has been designed in a very digestible way; as with a cookbook, if you follow the steps with care you will create beautiful dishes. Each chapter represents a week of the programme and is designed to help you use the least effort necessary to enjoy maximum rewards.

The programme is a carefully crafted interplay of both conscious and subconscious tools that will support you on your journey to optimal sleep.

The Sleep Well Programme is designed to take your hand and guide you gently through it from week to week so that your system is not overwhelmed. You need time to implement each new habit before moving to the next one. I truly hope that you can savour each week and luxuriate in the many pearls of wisdom offered. Remember, if you have been struggling with sleep issues on and off for years, it is going to take time to resolve them. I am much more interested in helping you transform your relationship with sleep for life rather than offering a momentary solution.

However, we all read books at our own pace. Some of us love to race ahead to the finish line and others prefer to dip in and out over a longer period. If you are the latter type, the structure of this book is already perfect for you! One chapter a week is manageable for most of us, no matter how busy you are. However, if you are (like me) someone who likes to eat books quickly and then digest them slowly by going back over pertinent points, then please feel free to read at the pace that suits you. The only non-negotiable is that you listen to each night-time audio for seven nights before you start the next one. I also highly recommend that having satisfied your curiosity, you go back and read each chapter again to correspond with the audio you are listening to. You deserve to give this everything you have, it is worth investing your precious time in. And the joy is that as your sleep quality inevitably improves, you will find the patience you require flows more easily.

Every week you will:

✦ Explore an aspect of the science and/or psychology of sleep – this engages the rational and conscious mind.

✦ Adopt a new practical lifestyle habit that is scientifically proven to improve the overall quality and effectiveness of your sleep. These habits are both manageable and flexible.

✦ Listen to the Sleep Well morning, rest (afternoon) and night-time audios every day. These are designed to fit into your current routine and will reinforce all your learnings on a subconscious level.

✦ ✦ ✦

The Sleep Well Formula

THE SLEEP WELL Formula is a reliable and solid key that opens the door to sleeping well. This formula is woven into the programme consciously as you read and subconsciously as you sleep. As I mentioned in the introduction, this formula was born, like many positive and creative discoveries, without force or pressure. The formula simplifies the process of going to sleep and getting back to sleep should you wake in the night. It operates on both a physiological and a psychological level.

The practical steps you apply each night engage the parasympathetic (rest and digest) nervous system, which is necessary for sleep to come to you. On a deeper psychological level, the formula cultivates the mindset required to stay asleep and you can rely on it, the way you would a loyal friend. Should you experience sleep challenges, applying the formula helps immediately. For example, if you have a bad night's sleep (for any reason from travel or hot flushes to a young child waking you up), the formula provides the certainty you need that you will sleep soundly the next night. The formula gives you the perspective needed to see that one broken night does not equate to two or three bad nights or indeed a lifetime of poor sleep.

The formula is crucial to your sleep success and, once rooted in your subconscious via the hypnotherapy audios, it will help you make an effortless transition from wakefulness into sleep. You will learn to apply it as you go to sleep and if you wake up in the middle of the night or early morning. Once you learn this formula and feel the benefit of it, it will become your steady anchor for sleep. No matter how stormy your life becomes, your innate ability to sleep will be securely embedded in your subconscious. This formula is effective for optimising the quality and depth of your sleep, and thus your life. With time, this becomes automatic, and you won't even know you are using it. Restorative, undisturbed and satisfying sleep becomes second nature.

Perhaps you are crying out at this stage, 'Fiona, will you share the formula?' I thank you for your patience; as you will see, this is a key strength when it comes to sleep and life. So, without further ado ... here it is.

Breathe + Imagine + Experience = Faith

I will explain each step and how it helps the body and mind to surrender to sleep. The most effective way to learn this formula is to experience it. I have made this really easy for you by embedding the formula into the night-time hypnotherapy audios. As you listen, the formula gradually becomes a default setting in your subconscious that allows you to effortlessly open the door to sleep.

STEP ONE: BREATHE

Sleep is not something you do or get; it is something you welcome into your body with deep, conscious breaths. The breath is the only part of the autonomic nervous system that remains under both your conscious and unconscious control.

> **Your breath is the bridge between your conscious and subconscious mind.**

It is because of this unique quality that you are in a position to communicate with your subconscious self. Most of the time you are breathing, you are doing so unconsciously; however, consciously leveraging your breathing to promote calmness and relaxation will change how you live and sleep.

I will share with you specific and evidence-based scientific breathing tools that, with practice, can help you to fall asleep within minutes and stay asleep. The hypnotherapy audios coupled with the yogic resting ritual included in this programme will change how you breathe. Your deeper and slower breathing will help you to reach a place of loving presence in which you will sleep peacefully.

STEP TWO: IMAGINE

The power of your imagination is the next piece of the formula. The image of your best-slept self needs to be cemented into your mind each day. Recall your intention and see it as being already realised. See the vitality in your eyes, feel the health and abundance of energy in your body and the confidence of regulated emotions. You are calm and positive, and life is flowing. Your imagination is a highly potent tool when you direct it to your advantage rather than your detriment.

> **This positive process has already begun; as you read these words and see the images I describe, you are becoming a better sleeper.**

You will direct your imagination to guide you into sleep. As you imagine yourself in the most beautiful, tranquil and relaxing places, using all your senses, sleep will come easily. One of the things I like to do and recommend you do too is to take a mental snapshot from your day of a beautiful scene. It could be your garden, your local park, a flower, a robin that you saw. Then, should you wake up in the middle of the night, use this image as your 'imagination step'. This is very effective as the picture is fresh in your mind and you can access it easily. It also encourages you to search the world for beauty each day.

STEP THREE: EXPERIENCE

Your imagination now creates your reality, and you will begin to experience solid, sound sleep night after night. You will know what it is like to wake up truly refreshed, with a clearer perspective and a more positive outlook. Once your sleep has improved you will begin to believe it's possible to sustain this new positive habit. From belief, you move into faith.

STEP FOUR: FAITH

As you experience better sleep, you will cultivate utter faith in the vision of your well-slept self. Faith goes beyond belief. It is something that once you have, you do not question. Faith is not dependent on knowing or striving towards certainty; it is about letting go completely and stepping into the unknown. Sleep is about surrendering to the power within you that is beyond your conscious control. Faith is unshakable. Having faith in yourself and your ability to sleep is the essence of a good life. Faith will quell any anxiety you once had about getting to sleep and staying asleep.

> **You will let go of fear and sleep easily, trusting
> it to take care of you, night after blissful night.**

Can you breathe? If you are reading this, you are breathing. You are alive and you do not question that process. You trust it. You have faith that your next breath will follow the last. Sleeping is no different from breathing: it naturally occurs. Faith is knowing something is true for you, whereas beliefs, both positive and negative, can be inherited from others. You were not born doubting your ability to sleep well; you picked up this doubt as a damaging belief. It is time to question it.

Unbeknownst to myself, before writing this book I too had unhelpful beliefs and doubted sleep. Now each night, no matter where I am, in order to fall sleep and stay asleep, I use this formula. It works. When it comes to faith and my relationship with sleep, I like to compare it to the relationship I have built over 20 years with my husband, Ciaran. I know that I can rely on him. Our bond is so close. It is not perfect, but I have faith in our relationship, and this allows me not to question our love for one another. Instead it gives me permission to enjoy it. The same is true of my ability to sleep well. I can rely on it. Do you have such a person in your own life who you trust and can depend on? If so, this is the faith I am referring to. Above all, cultivating faith in yourself is what matters most. Knowing that you can depend on yourself to make choices that serve you well is true liberation.

✦ ✦ ✦

Lifestyle Interventions and Healthy Habits

YOUR LIFESTYLE IS your health. The choices you make, from the food you eat to the people you spend time with, are the biggest indicators (outside infectious disease, genetic conditions, natural disasters and tragic accidents) that will determine how well and how long you live.

Lifestyle medicine is an evidence-based approach that focuses on using lifestyle interventions to prevent, manage and treat chronic diseases. Many health conditions, such as heart disease, type 2 diabetes, obesity, certain cancers, and mental health disorders, are hugely influenced by lifestyle factors such as diet, physical activity, stress, sleep and substance abuse.

The primary intention of lifestyle medicine is to uncover the root causes of disease by promoting healthy behaviours and modifying unhealthy ones. It emphasises the importance of lifestyle choices in improving overall health and well-being, rather than relying solely on medication or invasive procedures. Lifestyle medicine takes a holistic approach and is cognisant that treating one aspect of health in isolation from others is counterproductive. For example, when a doctor prescribes sleeping tablets that do not induce quality sleep and have the side effect of exhaustion, or you take pain medication for your head and it upsets your stomach.

Lifestyle medicine is helpful in alleviating up to 80 per cent of the world's most chronic health conditions.[2] One study on the impact of a Mediterranean-style diet on reducing the risk of heart disease recurrence showed that participants who ate more fruits, vegetables, whole grains, legumes, fish and olive oil had a 50–70 per cent lower risk of recurrent heart attacks and cardiac deaths compared to those following a standard low-fat diet.[3]

The emphasis on behavioural change and personal accountability for one's health is paramount for prevention rather than cure.

> **You are the active agent of living and ageing well. Why wait until you have a health condition to begin to take care of yourself?**

There are six pillars of lifestyle medicine and each one is vital to support a healthy body and mind and to prevent lifestyle diseases developing. However, sleep is the foundation and the other five need it to function. Each pillar is interconnected with the others; for example, if you are tired you will make unhealthy food choices and if you make unhealthy food choices it will impact your sleep.

If you consider the six components as a wheel, sleep is the hub and the remaining five are the spokes. Together, these spokes surround the hub of sleep, creating a balanced and interconnected wheel. The central placement of sleep reinforces the priority you now place on it and how it supports all the other behaviours in your life. Your well-slept self will naturally make healthier choices in your daily routine.

The six pillars are: sleep; exercise; nutrition (a whole-food, predominantly plant-based diet); stress management; avoiding risky substances, such as alcohol, smoking and narcotics; and positive social connections.

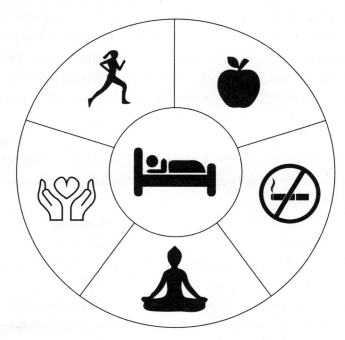

In an ideal setting, lifestyle medicine is practised by a multidisciplinary team of healthcare professionals, including doctors, consultants, nutritional therapists, personal trainers, psychologists, therapists and coaches. The idea is to empower the patient to know why they need to make better choices in order to prevent and manage chronic health conditions. Motivation is key. Many health services are under huge pressure and are not in a position to offer this type of care; however, you are in a position as a good sleeper to ensure you are doing all you can to give yourself the care that you deserve.

The eight habits you are beginning to build week by week cover the main components of the six pillars, with the emphasis always on optimising your sleep. As you sleep more soundly you will also move more, have a healthier diet and a calmer mind, lower your alcohol consumption and cultivate closer bonds with other people. If this sounds too good to be true, it isn't. Each spoke in the wheel is important and relies on the other spokes to do their parts. When one part of your life becomes healthier, it is logical that you will begin to make positive shifts in other areas. For example, if you are used to a regular sleep routine, you have more energy to exercise in the day. Each habit is realistic and often simply requires some gentle tweaks to your current lifestyle. The audios and my support are with you each step of the way.

✦ ✦ ✦

The Sleep Well Habits

DORIAN GRAY HAD his own secrets; but the rest of us mere mortals need to adopt daily routines that will help us to increase not just our lifespan but, more important, our health span. As one of my elderly neighbours

If I could get back my youth, I'd do anything in the world except get up early, take exercise or be respectable.

OSCAR WILDE,
THE PICTURE OF DORIAN GRAY

said, 'Life is short, but you can stretch it out.' To help you to introduce any new habit into your life, you need to make it easy. Habit stacking is a smart way to ensure you don't forget to do something you intended to do. This is the act of connecting a new habit with an existing one. Each week you are introduced to a new habit and in order to stack them correctly, you simply link the new one to the existing one. For example, the habit for Week One is to 'Go to sleep and wake up at roughly the same time every day' and the habit for Week Two is 'Create a "blissful hour" 60-minute bedtime routine.' To stack these habits, you need to make a strong connection between them. So, when you set your alarm for the morning, you also set a reminder to start getting ready for bed one hour before you intend to sleep. Habit stacking operates by optimising the brain circuitry that has already been established for a pre-existing habit to act as an internal reminder to introduce the new habit.

A great cue for stacking a new habit to is brushing your teeth. This habit is so well established in your morning and night-time routines and is now automatic, hence it is the perfect time and space to remind yourself of a new habit. For example, each time I brush my teeth at night, I remember to take my magnesium supplement. In the beginning, I had to consciously remember to take the supplement, but now the act of brushing my teeth reminds me. Find the tasks that you do every day at the same time and allow these to act as cues for you to introduce new positive habits into your life. You would be amazed at how many of these daily tasks you already do routinely, for example feeding the dog, putting out the bins, and so on.

Another helpful way to introduce a new habit is to remind yourself before you go to sleep at night of your intention for the next morning. For example, if you want to get out into the light as soon as you wake, say out loud or write, 'When I wake up in the morning, I am getting out into the natural light or maximising the artificial lights in my home.' Have your clothes and runners ready and waiting for you or your LED light fully charged.

You learn to match your environment with your intention.

It is important to keep in mind as you work through the eight habits that a good night's sleep begins as soon as you open your eyes. It is likely that you are already practising some of the eight habits and others will be new to you. Each habit is backed up with solid sleep science and it is important that you understand why they are so beneficial to your well-being. When you can see the logic of the habits and feel the mental, physical and emotional rewards they offer, your motivation to implement them will increase.

The weekly night-time hypnotherapy audios that you are listening to are designed to consistently reinforce, on a subconscious level, your commitment to sleeping well. It may surprise you to notice how effortlessly you begin to adopt the habits. Like a well-loved pet, you won't be able to imagine life without them. The benefits you feel will ensure that with time they become automatic. We are pleasure-seeking creatures, and the pleasure of waking up refreshed and having positive energy throughout your day becomes a catalyst for sustainable change.

The eight habits are not designed to be rigid or for you to use as a means to be hard on yourself when they are less than perfect. You need to move through each habit at your own pace and in your own time. Each of the habits is based on cutting-edge sleep science that I practise myself and have recommended to countless clients. There are days when I do all of them and days when I do just one or two. Context matters, and your best is always enough. In each chapter, I share how they work for me, to give you some support for the habits you may find challenging. Positive habits become rewarding rituals that provide a sense of peace and security. Each habit is carefully designed to enhance your lifestyle, not to curtail it.

In terms of importance, each habit has its significant role to play, and therefore they are all equal. It is never just one thing that contributes to a good life or sleep; it is a combination of different elements that come together. You will know which factors work for you. Regardless of which habits resonate with you most, what matters is that you cultivate a balanced nervous system during both the day and night. The eight habits provide you with the power and tools to navigate your state of arousal – to be alert and relaxed during periods of activity in the day and to be calm when you rest and sleep.

I am here to remind you that the most important thing is to let go of perfection and striving. If one day life gets in the way of practising any of the habits, step in and take back control the next day. Be gentle – but firm – with yourself. Self-compassion is not self-pity, and holding yourself accountable to your best-slept self is vital.

The eight positive sleep habits provide a lifetime reference point for you. At first, as with any new skill, this can seem like a lot to take on. Fret not, each habit is reinforced in your night-time audios, so the message is received on a subconscious level. You are not relying on willpower. The important thing is not to try to do too much too soon.

Habit change works best in small steps and by acknowledging each tiny success and then continuing.

The common denominators with all sleep obstacles are stress and anxiety, so the logical thing to do is to reduce the stress reaction. The Sleep Well Programme tackles this problem in a highly effective way by helping you to slow down your thoughts and at the same time cultivating three key strengths that will optimise your sleep and elevate your life.

✦ ✦ ✦

The Three Sleep Strengths

WHAT IS UNIQUE about this programme is that as your sleep slowly improves you are simultaneously reprogramming your brain with three core strengths for sleep and life.

The strengths of presence, patience and peace have been specifically chosen to help you to sleep peacefully and live fully. In your night-time audios these strengths are introduced, repeated and reinforced as you drift to sleep. The last three weeks of this course are dedicated to each strength in turn, but from the first night you listen, the three sleep strengths are already taking root in your malleable subconscious mind. As the strengths become more deeply ingrained in your subconscious, your ability to sleep longer and deeper grows. You become the active agent for positive shifts in your waking world as you sleep. I have identified these three strengths as key to sleep, but they are also central to a life well lived. They literally give you the strength to implement the habits slowly and to pick yourself up if you have a night of broken sleep and struggle the next day. When you are present, patient and peaceful, you are free to do your best without any internal judgement.

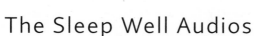

The Sleep Well Audios

AS YOU KNOW, this book works on a practical and a psychological level. It also works on a conscious and a subconscious level. The audios are designed to bring the Law of Least Effort into practice.

Start tonight, if you haven't already done so, to listen to the Sleep Well audios. You can access these audios with the passcode ISLEEPWELL on www.thepositivehabit.com.

This part is where you can lie back and do absolutely nothing and allow your entire being to radiate as you sleep. The phrase 'neurons that wire together fire together' was coined by Dr Carla Shatz and refers to the strength of the connection between two neurons when they are repeatedly activated. Neurons transmit information to each other through chemical and electrical signals via the synaptic connections in your brain. You are establishing a new neural network that represents your faith in your ability to maintain good sleep each time you listen to your hypnotherapy audios.

However, the purpose of your hypnotherapy sleep time audios is twofold. The first is to improve your overall sleep quality. The relaxation process activates your parasympathetic nervous system and helps you glide from a conscious state (the thinking mind) into the subconscious (the imagination).

The second benefit is enhancing your emotional well-being (through positive suggestions) as you sleep. Martin Seligman, the founder of Positive Psychology, defines emotional well-being as 'The experience of positive emotions such as contentment, joy, and happiness, the absence of negative emotions, and the sense of life being meaningful and fulfilling.'

Negative emotions play an essential role in helping you to understand yourself and should never be dismissed; however, as you go to sleep, you clearly do not want to be in a state of stress that activates your nervous system.

You are now in a positive relationship with sleep.

It is one of mutual respect, and as you prioritise sleep it rewards you with increased health and vitality and a feeling of emotional balance.

It is essential you listen to the instructions for the audios. They will help you to optimise your listening and relaxing experience. My voice will create a Pavlovian conditioning effect for going to sleep. Often listeners are asleep within the first couple of minutes of hearing my voice. The audios are not only effective at helping you to get to sleep and stay asleep, but they also increase the overall quality and depth of your sleep, so you awaken more refreshed. Continuing to listen each night is a wonderful means of sustaining positive neuroplastic change. Many of my clients , like Fionnuala, whom you met earlier, use these audios as tools for life. Others dip in and out of them as needed. The audios can be helpful for both acute (short-term) and chronic stress. This can range from a minor disruption such as changes in your environment, like travel or holidays, or the lead-up to an important presentation or social occasion, to more serious issues, for example if you are suffering grief or a diagnosis of ill health. You can be assured of a good night's sleep, no matter what is going on in your life.

The night-time audios use the Sleep Well Formula as their core focus, and the more often you listen, the more you will learn how to apply the formula effortlessly. Self-hypnosis occurs when you are able to induce the same state of relaxation yourself by using the steps in the formula without any need to turn on or listen to the audios. The three sleep strengths are gradually introduced into the audios each week (and explored fully in Weeks 6,7 and 8), which will help you to establish the habit of sleeping well and living fully.

It is imperative that you listen for a minimum of eight weeks. Start today if you haven't already. To establish a new habit, the reward of feeling the benefits of this behaviour is crucial to your success. Recall the image of your well-slept self and let that guide you.

Your Sleep Well audios are designed to help you at key stages during the day.

✦ The morning meditation is ten minutes long.

✦ The afternoon or evening rest ritual is seven minutes long.

✦ The night-time hypnotherapy audios are approximately 25 minutes, but since you listen to them in bed they do not require any extra time from your day. Most people are asleep within minutes. Please note it is also possible to listen to the night-time audios as part of a longer afternoon nap routine. I do this often, and it primes me to sleep well at night.

I have also included a 4,7,8 breathing protocol for you to practise, and it is excellent for calming you if you feel overwhelmed during the day or for returning to sleep if you wake at any stage in the night.

A NOTE ABOUT DEVICES

Sleep scientists advise you to keep your phone out of the bedroom completely, and for good reasons. First of all, the blue light from the screen interrupts your circadian rhythm, and second, giving in to the temptation to check apps, emails, texts, etc. increases levels of dopamine and cortisol right at the time of day that you need to be winding down, not up. However, for the purpose of listening to your Sleep Well night-time audio, we have a rather paradoxical situation that requires, I will admit, a very enlightened approach.

Do you have a hammer in your home? I imagine you do. You could use it to hang up a picture, fix a broken chair, destroy something, or even hurt yourself or another. The hammer is just a tool, and it is up to you how you use it. Your phone is the same. You can use it to enhance your life or deplete it.

The phone has become a magnet that pulls your attention towards it, often promising pleasure and leaving you numb. I am sure you can relate to the fatigue, disconnection and anxiety that come from getting lost in your phone. British-Swiss writer and journalist Johann Hari's latest book, *Stolen Focus: Why You Can't Pay Attention*, wants Big Tech to take responsibility for the way their products hijack our attention with algorithms that are designed to grab us and keep us mindlessly scrolling. He argues that people need to stop blaming themselves for their tech addictions.

People who work in Big Tech are the first ones to implement boundaries between themselves and their smartphones. A former strategist for Google once asked a group of hundreds of leading tech designers, 'How many of you want to live in the world you are designing?' There was silence in the room. People looked around them. Nobody put up their hand. In his book, Hari states, 'Your attention didn't collapse, it was stolen.'[4]

The smartphone is pretty clever, but it is not just a phone. In fact, voice-calling is one of its least popular features. According to a 2018 survey by Deloitte, only 31 per cent of smartphone users in the United States use their phones to make calls on a daily basis, compared to 49 per cent who use messaging apps and 89 per cent who use social media.[5]

The key is that you choose how to use the device – rather than it using you. It is a torch, a camera, a GPS, a clock, a timer and, for this purpose, an audio player. I believe the benefits of listening to your audio outweigh the ill effects of having your phone in your bedroom – but only when you are its master and not its servant. **It must be there for the sole purpose of using it to listen to the hypnotherapy audios.**

While we wait for Big Tech to change its ways, you need to take the situation into your own hands. Now is the time for you to take back what was stolen from you. You are in control and your device is in safe hands. Follow these guidelines to listen to your audios on your smartphone with minimal disruption and maximum benefit. I practise these myself, and, after time, they require no effort.

✦ Switch your phone to Night Shift mode to automatically dim down its light from two hours before you go to bed until you wake up.

✦ Select the audio you wish to listen to that night and have it ready, so it is just one click away.

- Stay off your phone for two hours before bed.

- Turn off ALL your notifications. (I recommend you also do this during the day.)

- After you select your night-time audio, refrain from checking any other apps.

- Use wireless headphones, if you have them, and keep your phone on the other side of or even just outside your bedroom. If you don't have wireless headphones, keep the phone facing down. (Please note that you should always listen to your audio in stereo.)

If you find the above steps too challenging to begin with and the temptation to scroll too great, be patient and remember that you can also use the night-time hypnotherapy audios as a relaxing meditation before you go to bed. You can then enter your room primed for sleep – just make sure to keep the lights dim. You need to find what works best for YOU.

If you are on the other end of the scale and do not have a smartphone, perhaps you could ask someone to help you download the tracks to your computer or tablet and listen from there.

MANUALLY TRACK YOUR SLEEP

Do you wear a digital sleep tracker? If so, do you find it helps or hinders your relationship with sleep? Perhaps you have found it useful. But for many people who worry about their sleep, it simply intensifies their concern. A study published in the *Journal of Health Psychology* found that people experienced anxiety related to the accuracy and interpretation of their self-tracking data, noting that 'the act of measuring and monitoring itself can become a source of anxiety'.[6] Often people become fixated on the amount of time they spent in the various stages of sleep.

> **Monitoring sleep in this way is akin to a person who is worried about their weight constantly stepping on and off the scales.**

The checking becomes compulsive, and if the number is not 'right' then a feeling of failure ensues, and with it comes low self-esteem. If you see a less-than-perfect amount of time spent in deep sleep or REM, it can induce thoughts like 'I'm not even good at sleeping.' But you are as good a sleeper as anyone else – remember that.

In addition, the science is still not clear on how accurate the data from sleep-tracking devices is. You could be fretting about nothing and in fact making the situation much worse than it originally was. Dr Matthew Walker, previously mentioned, notes that the only way to get 100 per cent accuracy in evaluating the effectiveness of your sleep is by going into a sleep lab, which is clearly not accessible to most of us. In addition, Walker states that most digital trackers on the market are only 60 per cent accurate, as they often make major errors in the amount of time spent in REM and deep sleep. I recommend that, for now, you manually track your sleep.

To do this, you don't need any devices. Simply observe how you feel. You won't get the specific numbers and minutes that you spent in the various stages of sleep, but you will connect to your body and evaluate for yourself your energy levels, your emotional state, and your ability to recall information. You will work closely with your internal clock and create intimacy and trust with yourself that no device can ever deliver. You will begin to rely on your own internal system and judge for yourself how you feel as you rest more, sleep peacefully and grow your three core sleep strengths.

Build Your Sleep Well Habits

IT IS TIME to introduce you to your first Sleep Well habit of going to sleep and waking up at roughly the same time every day. This very instrumental change is the first you need to make. You could very well be doing this already, and if so, wonderful. If not, establishing a regular routine for going to sleep and waking up is the foundation for effective, reliable sleep. The word 'roughly' is important here – the routine is not rigid.

HABIT ONE

Go to sleep and wake up at roughly the same time every day.

THE BODY RESPONDS to routine, and routine is fundamental for maximising the quality of your sleep. Go to sleep and rise at roughly the same time each day, including weekends and holidays. This may sound boring, yet there is nothing mundane about feeling full of life and energy.

> If you have good habits, time becomes your ally. All you need is patience.
>
> JAMES CLEAR

There are two main types of sleep: rapid eye movement (REM) and non-rapid eye movement (NREM). Within NREM, there are three different stages and each one plays a pivotal role. Each sleep cycle lasts roughly 90 minutes, and you need five of these each night. When you multiply five by 90 minutes, you get 450 minutes, which is seven and a half hours, the minimum sleep time needed by adults. The eight-hour sleep recommendation includes extra time to compensate for the time it takes you to go to sleep and any interruptions you may have through the night, for example going to the bathroom.

To calculate the time you need to be going to sleep, work back eight hours from when you need to get up for work or wish to rise. So, for example, if you wish to wake up at 7 a.m., you need to be asleep by 11 p.m. In order to be asleep by 11 p.m., you need to begin to unwind at 10 p.m. This is further explained in Habit Two – 'Create a "blissful hour" 60-minute bedtime routine'.

Even if you have complete autonomy over your waking time, get into the habit of rising at roughly the same time seven days a week. The weekend is a concept of the mind and a construct of civilisation rather than nature.

Your body has its own clock that will answer to nothing but nature.

A growing body of research indicates that the first four hours of sleep are the most important in terms of the benefits for our brain's capacity to process and consolidate memories.[7] The hours before midnight are particularly effective for this. The protein synthesis that builds memories in our brain happens in these earlier cycles of sleep. If you have learned something new during the day, the earlier REM sleep cycles you enter are much more likely to cement that information for you than the later dream cycles. The latest sleep science indicates that when you miss the earlier sleep cycles by going to bed later than you normally would, you miss the opportunity for both of the benefits of processing and consolidating memories to occur.

Imagine you have a meeting in a different city, and you miss the train you needed to get to arrive on time. You can catch a later train, but the meeting has already started and you have missed the main insights. The human growth hormone (HGH) is connected to the body's master biological clock. HGH is released at the same time each night. Like the train pulling out of the station, it doesn't wait. So, for example, if you normally go to sleep at 11 p.m. but stay awake until 1 a.m. because of a social occasion, you lose two hours of this quality sleep and you can't get it back. This explains why you are less refreshed the day after you break your routine and your mind will be foggier, even though you might have had the same amount of sleep.

According to Dr Gina Poe, who specialises in the area of memory consolidation and sleep at the UCLA Brain Research Institute, 'One of the best markers of good neurological health when we get older is consistent bedtimes.' A rigid routine doesn't sound terribly exciting or conducive to a wild social life; however, if you are going to compromise your routine, make sure it is worth it! When you do break your routine, keep any changes to your wake-up time to a maximum of one hour and stick to the same eating schedule. Don't try to compensate with a long lie-in, as this is counterproductive. Instead, opt for a short nap or rest. This is expanded on in Habit Seven: 'Take time to rest every day in the middle of your day'.

What this Looks Like for Me
I rise early. I love the fresh start of an early morning. My energy and focus are at optimal levels. I often organise social events

earlier in the evening, and I avoid booking early or late flights when I can. But sometimes the joy of socialising late, getting a night-time flight or picking up my son from a party is more than worth it. I also tend to shift seasonally, going to bed slightly later and rising later in the summer months. When I do go to bed later, I naturally wake at the same time as usual and compensate with a nap. Within a day, I'm back on track.

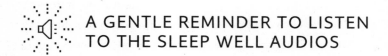

A GENTLE REMINDER TO LISTEN TO THE SLEEP WELL AUDIOS

You can access these audios for FREE with the passcode ISLEEPWELL on www.thepositivehabit.com.

Please remember to listen to the instructions for listening to guarantee maximum benefits.

MORNING MEDITATION

Please listen each morning to 'Start Your Day in Stillness – Intention-Setting Morning Meditation' to slow down your thoughts before the day commences.

AFTERNOON OR EVENING REST RITUAL

Please listen to 'Seven-Minute Rest Ritual' each afternoon and/or evening.

NIGHT-TIME HYPNOTHERAPY – WEEK ONE: HABIT ONE

This is the most important track to listen to. Each week there are new subconscious suggestions to help to reinforce the corresponding weekly habit and the following key insights.

To Get Back to Sleep if You Wake Up

You can listen to your night-time audio again, if necessary, but with time you will not need to do this. The Sleep Well Formula (Breathe + Imagine + Experience = Faith), which you are learning on a subconscious level every time you listen to your weekly audios, will become automatic. Please also listen to the '4, 7, 8 Breathing' audio and train yourself to do this in the middle of the night should you awaken.

THE 4, 7, 8 BREATHING TECHNIQUE

The 4, 7, 8 breathing technique was developed by Dr Andrew Weil and is based on yogi-controlled breathing. It has been proven to help people fall asleep more quickly and I recommend practising it if you wake in a lighter phase of sleep.

Weil points out that the benefits accumulate over time, that within four weeks of practising four cycles twice a day, it becomes a stress reduction tool that you can utilise when you feel triggered by a situation or person to help you to move from reacting to responding.

This technique and other breathing protocols are also a way to interrupt unhealthy habitual patterns of behaviour such as comfort eating, drinking or smoking. When you feel a craving for something you can use this technique to calm your nervous system and let the craving pass.

After two or three months of continued practice there are very significant changes that happen on a physiological level: your heart rate and blood pressure lower, your digestion improves, and it is a very powerful tool to release anxiety and stress. The more you practise, the slower and deeper your breath becomes. Please listen and practise every day, especially if you enter a lighter phase of sleep in the night or early morning. You will be back to sleep quickly.

THE GOLDEN KEY INSIGHTS FROM WEEK ONE: YOUR DECISION TO SLEEP WELL

✦ You have a clear image of yourself one year from now looking back at you from a mirror. You can see your best-slept self, healthy, energised and fully awake to the wonder of the world.

✦ You are in a relationship with sleep and have decided to prioritise it so that you can welcome it each night.

✦ You have a clear picture of your sleep habits as they stand and you will return to the sleep surveys and the 'How Present are You?' quiz on p. 33 at the end of the eight-week programme.

✦ The Law of Least Effort will help you to learn the Sleep Well Formula: Breathe + Imagine + Experience = Faith. Each time you listen to your night-time audio, the formula is being reinforced so you do not have to actively recall it.

✦ The six pillars of lifestyle medicine are all important for your health and longevity, but sleep is the foundation for the other five.

✦ Habit One is 'Go to sleep and wake up at roughly the same time every day.'

To maximise the benefits of this programme, I encourage you not to begin reading Week Two until you have listened to the 'Week One: Habit One' night-time audio for a minimum of seven nights in total.

I hope you are enjoying your first week's audios. Remember, if you miss a night or day of listening to your audios or getting to bed or rising at the same time, it is absolutely fine. Habits take time to form, so be patient with yourself and acknowledge your progress. You are reading this and taking positive action to improve your sleep – well done.

YOUR SLEEP STORY

We are the stories we tell ourselves.

JOAN DIDION

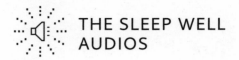

THE SLEEP WELL AUDIOS

All audios are available to download on www.thepositivehabit.com with the password ISLEEPWELL.

Please listen to the short instructional audio track 'Instructions', if you haven't already done so. It will provide you with an overview of how to listen to your hypnotherapy audios every day.

✦ Tonight, please start listening to 'Week Two: Habit Two' of the Sleep Well audios. Please listen to this audio for a minimum of seven nights. Please do not skip ahead to Week Three until you have listened for a full seven days.

✦ Please also continue to listen to your morning meditation and your rest ritual tracks each day.

✦ ✦ ✦

Measure Your Sleep

BEFORE YOU BEGIN Week Two of the Sleep Well Programme, please take a moment to rate your sleep. On a scale of 0 to 10, how well have you slept in the last week? (0 is 'terribly' and 10 is 'very well'.) Please use the image on the opposite page to mark where you feel you are on this scale.

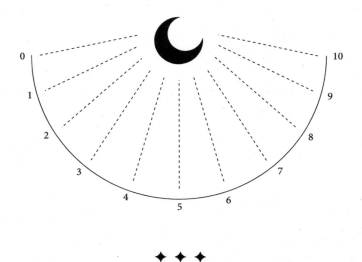

✦ ✦ ✦

Welcome to Week Two

MANY PEOPLE FEEL an almost immediate benefit of listening to the audios and shifting their mindset towards sleep in as short a period as a week. If this is you, wonderful. If not, no problem – the most important thing is to keep going and the faith will come. You will make the progress you need in your own way, in your own time. Sleep is definitely not a competitive sport.

This week you are going to learn about the neuroscience of what happens when you go to sleep. You will explore the importance of letting go so that you can sleep. You will look at how feeling safe at a biological level is essential for you to surrender into sweet slumber. You will complete the very worthwhile exercise of writing your own sleep story, starting from when you were a child. This can be very illuminating and something most of us never take the time to do. Once you have written this you will begin to question some of the conditioned negative beliefs you may have about how you rate yourself as a sleeper.

This week's habit is one of my favourites. It turns bedtime into something you genuinely look forward to. Habit Two, 'Create a "blissful hour" 60-minute bedtime routine', is exactly that: pure bliss.

◆ ◆ ◆

The Scientific Door to Sleep

DURING THE SPANISH flu pandemic that raged across Europe just after the end of World War I, Austrian neurologist Constantin von Economo discovered something spectacular.[8] He studied two types of flu patients: the first type fell into a deep lethargy or coma before dying; the second type did not sleep at all before eventually surrendering to death. Von Economo conducted autopsies on the two different types of patients' brains and discovered that they had different types of lesions. In the brains of the patients who had slept before they died, he found damage in the posterior hypothalamus, the upper part of the midbrain. Von Economo coined the term 'wakefulness centre' to refer to the part of the brain that maintains wakefulness. The patients who had not been able to sleep before dying had lesions in the preoptic area of the anterior hypothalamus, and this part came to be known as the 'sleep centre'.

This seminal work enabled scientists who conducted autopsies on people who died after being in a coma to discover that the brain-stem plays a significant role in wakefulness. They learned that there are two major circuits in the brainstem that interact with one another to induce either sleep or wakefulness. This interaction is controlled by the body's internal clock. Think of this interaction as the door that opens and closes between the two states. You have a handle just at the base of your brainstem that you can open night after night.

✦ ✦ ✦

How Do You Open the Door?

IN THE SLEEP Well hypnotherapy audios, I use the metaphor of the door to sleep, and for a door, you need a key. This key is gold, and it can't be lost. When you cross the threshold from wakefulness to sleep, you shut down your external world and enter an internal place of peace and sleep. Your breath, coupled with visualisation, is the key that opens this door. Once you close the door, the roles you play and the responsibilities you have all melt away. You step away from worries, to-do lists and the challenges of your external world.

When you first walk through the door of wakefulness to sleep, you are in a hallway or corridor, and this is a place of gentle transition from one level of consciousness to another. As you relinquish the future and the past, and move towards now, you begin to move into an even deeper dimension that goes beyond time and space. There is no past or future as you slip in and out of awareness. Your mind in this phase will begin to drift into the slow theta brainwave state. We will explore this more in Week Four. Theta brainwave is common in hypnosis and guided meditations that encourage you to relax and use your imagination. It is a highly creative state in which random images and thoughts emerge.

In order to fall asleep, you simply need to allow yourself to drift and to enjoy the process of surrendering. As you place all your attention on my voice, I am guiding you towards the door and making this transition seamless.

The habits ensure that your door is ready to be opened. Faith – that unshakable knowing that you are capable of sleeping peacefully – is, as you know, at the heart of your ability to sleep well. Your overall mindset is also imperative and the first principle to nudge the door open is to learn to let go.

Radical Surrendering

TARA BRACH, AMERICAN psychologist, author and Buddhist meditation teacher, tells the story of a man who falls off the edge of a cliff and calls out to God.

'Are you there?'

A booming voice from the sky says, 'YES.'

The man says, 'God, can you help me? I'll do anything.'

God says, 'JUST LET GO.'

The man says, 'Is there anybody else there?'

The last thing we want to do is let go, to be open to the unknown. Why are you so afraid to let go? Like the man on the cliff, you don't feel safe to do so. Yet, unlike the man, you are *not* on a cliff. You can only let go when you feel safe. This safety comes from within, and once you feel this in every cell of your being, you will live and sleep like you have never done before. John O'Donohue, Irish poet and priest, once said, 'There is a place inside all of us that has never been wounded.' In order to go to sleep, you need to connect to this place. I will help, and sleep will help. It is there, inside you, inside all of us. Awakening your best-slept self is a process that can only happen when you feel secure.

Try this simple thought experiment with me now: take a look around the space you are in. If you are at home, do you feel secure? Is the building you are in safely built? Is it likely to fall down? Are any potential bombs going to fall? Is anyone likely to burst in and attack you? I do hope these things are not a concern for you, and if they are a possibility, it is understandable that you may find it hard to let go of control at night. However, if you are genuinely safe, can you recall a time when you didn't feel as physically safe? Perhaps you spent a night alone in an old country house or were out camping in the woods and heard animal noises from the bushes.

Now spend a moment reflecting on a situation at work or in your personal life that you find difficult. Perhaps you are worried about a family member, finances or a relationship conflict, or maybe you are overwhelmed due to unrealistic pressure put on you at work. Do you notice that the feeling of being unsafe physically is the same in your body? When you think about a psychological threat, the body interprets it in the same way as a physical one. It becomes tense and alert – not a state that is conducive to sleep. In both of these scenarios, your amygdala (also known as the fear centre of the brain), a small almond-shaped structure located in the medial temporal lobe of your brain, is firing up and sending messages to your nervous system to release cortisol and adrenaline.

✦ ✦ ✦

What Will Help You to Feel Safe?

SOAK IN YOUR environment and allow yourself to acknowledge that you are physically safe. The building you are in is unlikely to fall down, the house is secure, and you are, I hope, in a safe neighbourhood. If these things are not the case, consider what you can do, no matter how small, to take charge of the situation. If the external threats are out of your control, then rest assured that these principles will still help you. In fact, you need them more than anyone.

The following two core psychological ingredients will strengthen your feeling of safety.

A CLEAR CONSCIENCE

Your conscience is your moral compass and when it is not clear, it will cause you distress. Your conscience carries guilt for behaviours that you feel ashamed of. When it comes to letting go and allowing the door to sleep to open, it is essential that you know the difference between necessary guilt and unnecessary shame. Necessary guilt is when you have due cause for remorse: you have hurt someone, intentionally or otherwise. If you have reason to feel guilty for past behaviours, it is important to take responsibility, be accountable and forgive yourself before you can let the guilt go.

Forgiveness of the self or others is not something that comes easily to many of us. I find it helpful to remember that we can only operate at our level of consciousnesses at the time of the action. This does not condone wrongdoing, but it does help me to be kinder to my younger self and others.

Unnecessary shame is much more common and presents as being very hard on yourself for no valid reason, for example when you have made a genuine mistake or feel shame about the behaviour of a family member. It can also arise in feeling not good enough as a parent or a daughter, partner, etc. In a work situation, it can manifest as impostor syndrome, where you may feel you are not skilled or educated enough to do your job. That one day you will be found out and asked to leave. Many people in high-level positions feel this.

TRUST IN YOUR INNATE ABILITY TO SLEEP

There is a story of a beggar who had been sitting on the side of the road for over thirty years. One day, when he was sitting in his usual spot on the side of the road and hoping someone would give him money, he saw a stranger walking by. The beggar asked the man for some spare change.

The man responded, 'I don't have any, but what is that you are sitting on?'

'Just an empty box,' replied the beggar.

'Have you ever looked inside?' the man said.

'There is no point. It is empty.'

'Have a look,' said the man encouragingly. 'You never know what you will find.'

The beggar rather reluctantly got up and opened the lid with some difficulty, and to his complete astonishment, he saw the box was filled with gold.

It is time to give yourself back the most precious gift of life – sleep. I want to highlight that you are giving yourself back something you have had all along. You are the beggar (no offence) and I am the stranger. I am helping you to open your own box of gold: sleep.

You already know how to sleep peacefully; you have just forgotten.

Your ability to sleep is innate. Inborn behaviours, such as sleeping, feeding, foraging, reproductive behaviours and protective responses, are all crucial to survival. You can rely on them to keep you alive.[9] Your circadian rhythm is part of your autonomic nervous system, which is an involuntary system and one that is out of your conscious control, hence trusting the process is essential.

Observe babies and toddlers: they do not doubt their ability to sleep. Infants are our greatest teachers of the art of letting go once their needs are met. On a busy and noisy train or bus, you are likely to see a baby or young child sound asleep. A baby requires both physical and psychological needs to be met in order to go to sleep. You are no different. Like happiness, sleep is within you.

✦ ✦ ✦

Remembering Your Sleep Story

ARIANNA HUFFINGTON, AUTHOR of *The Sleep Revolution*, explains how, despite being taught by her mother as a child in Athens to honour sleep, she found herself many years later caught up in America's corporate culture, which saw sleeping as a waste of time.[10] Arianna was, like many of her generation, convinced that people who forgo sleep to meet deadlines are more successful. For many people caught in this toxic culture, it is often the ultimate deadline of their own funeral that they are hurtling towards. Arianna tells the story in her book that one day, having only slept for three to four hours, she collapsed from exhaustion in her New York apartment. Her sister Agapi heard the fall and rushed in to see her lying in a pool of blood. Arianna had broken her cheekbone and was rushed to hospital. Like many parents, she had been trying to be everything to everyone, looking after her children during the day and running a business at night. Arianna left no space in her life for quality sleep, and her body simply gave out.

It was not that she could not sleep; she was choosing not to. She believed that the time she spent asleep was a waste and that she needed to use this time to work. It was returning to her roots and remembering how her mother ensured a peaceful and loving environment for Arianna and her sister to sleep in that helped. She recalled that in her childhood 'there was a respect for sleep as an integral part of life'.

Sleeping well is innate, but you can lose the skill depending on your own personal sleep story, beginning in your childhood. No matter what state of health your relationship with sleep is in now, it is never too late to transform it. I have worked with clients in their seventies and eighties and helped them to feel calmer during the day so that they can sleep more peacefully at night. Your door may have rusty hinges, but you do have a door, and together, with patience and love, we are gently reopening it. Knowing which chronotype you are will help us on our journey.

Which Chronotype Are You?

A BEAR, A lion, a wolf or a dolphin? A chronotype is your own personal predetermined rhythm that influences whether you prefer to rise early or burn the midnight oil. Your chronotype is part of your sleep story and will help you understand how your sleeping patterns have changed over the phases of your life.

Identifying your innate sleep–wake cycle is very beneficial in optimising the quality of your sleep, your overall energy levels and also the best times to consume caffeine, eat, exercise and even have sex.

Many people who report not feeling refreshed despite getting eight hours of sleep could be unwittingly working against their chronotype. This is an unfortunate side effect for many people who are forced to adapt to fit in with the demands of society, for example, starting school or work early if you are a night owl.

There are four chronotypes, according to Dr Michael Breus, clinical psychologist, sleep specialist and author of the groundbreaking book *The Power of When*. Can you identify which one you are?

BEAR

You are the most common type (approx. 55 per cent of people) and you sit in a healthy place between an early bird and a night owl. The 9–5 working day suits you perfectly, as your sleep–wake cycle is directly aligned with sunrise and sunset. Your energy and productivity levels peak before noon and then progressively begin to dip in the afternoon. You go to bed relatively early but not so early that you don't have the capacity for a social life at night.

LION

You are the quintessential early bird, rising at dawn. You like to get up and straight into your to-do list without delay. You value exercise and have good levels of energy spread throughout the day. Early rising makes a social life difficult; you are the type who will be booking the restaurant for 6 p.m. and looking for a taxi by 8 p.m. to get home to wind down in the early evening so that you are asleep by 9 or 10 p.m.

WOLF

You are more commonly known as the night owl. You really don't like going to bed early. You come alive after dark and find this time is when you are most creative and focused. You are also likely to be the last person to leave a party. You struggle with getting up in the morning and find it difficult to engage with the world for a few hours. Unfortunately for you, this is the toughest type to be in the working environment or at school.

DOLPHIN

You have an erratic schedule, and you show lion tendencies; however, your sleep is so poor at night that you will struggle to rise, and your energy levels will dip a lot during the day. You will most likely suffer from sleep anxiety and are unsure of how to improve your schedule. You find the slightest noise wakes you up. You are highly sensitive to your sleeping environment, you don't like to sleep in new places and you find travel a challenge. On the positive side, you do tend to have good energy and productivity levels between 10 a.m. and 2 p.m. each day.

To help you further identify your chronotype, I recommend that you take the quiz designed by Dr Breus on his site, sleepdoctor.com.

I am a lion on the cusp of a bear, which I love, but which presents a challenge when socialising after midnight. Once you have identified your chronotype, the question you might have is can you change it? It is possible to tweak it with your lifestyle choices to help you become more of a morning person, and many people do successfully do this. As a wolf, getting up early is more difficult to change, but with commitment, it is possible to begin by slowly bringing bedtime earlier each night. I become more of a bear in the summer months, going to bed later and rising later.

As you reflect on your life, you will see that at different times you have had different chronotypes. This is known as your sleep chronology and usually follows this pattern:

As a baby you were a lion, loving nothing more than waking the house up at 5 a.m. As a toddler and young child you became a bear, and as a teenager you would most likely have been a wolf, loving to stay up late and to sleep in. From the age of twenty or so, the body sets into one of the four chronotypes for approximately forty years. Then you begin to go backwards: you slowly return to being a lion. Notice how many older people like to eat early and go to bed early.

If you feel you don't fit into any of these categories, it is likely you are suffering from insomnia and stuck in the dolphin stage, which leads to confusion and exhaustion. (This is discussed further in Week 5, Embrace the Challenges.) Knowing your chronotype will help determine the times you choose for your Habit One ('Go to sleep and wake up at roughly the same time every day').

Before you write your sleep story, I would like to share my own. I hope it inspires you, like Fionnuala's in Week One, to see that improving your sleep is something we can all do.

✦ ✦ ✦

My Sleep Story

WHEN I WAS seven years old, I was an extremely happy, determined little human, friendly and full of laughter, fun and ideas. I loved my bed; it was my special place. I would make my bed as soon as I woke up early every morning, full of positive energy and excited for the day ahead. I shared a room with my beautiful big sister. I was on the bottom bunk and always felt very safe in the knowledge that she was above me, looking out for me. I slept soundly, like a baby.

Ironically, I have been told that I was not a good sleeper as a baby. I had colic and screamed all the time. My parents tell tales of driving me around in the car until I fell asleep. When I was a toddler, my family and I went to live in Greece. It was an epic adventure. We travelled from island to island looking for a home. We slept in different rooms all the time and sometimes on boats or beaches. I slept through it all. I learnt to take sleep where and when I could get it.

'You can sleep when you are dead.' You may have heard this phrase. My mother used to say it to me when I complained of being tired. I recall her saying it to me in Athens one night, as she tried her best to help me to stay awake during an all-nighter travelling from Dublin to the Cycladic island of Paros.

In my mother's defence, the science wasn't clear in the nineteen-eighties. The post-war generation generally held the opinion that sleep was necessary but unproductive. It should be kept to a minimum and too much of it was equated to being lazy or weak. This conviction manifested due to the rise of industrialisation and the emphasis on economic success. The view that sleep was a luxury was widespread. Mercifully, this belief is changing, and people now at least know the theory of why we need to sleep. For many, though, the idea remains that rest and naps result in lethargy.

My childhood ended abruptly at about twelve years old, and in my teenage years and young adulthood, my emotional landscape changed for various reasons, including grief and trauma. I now understand that I was suffering from chronic anxiety. My emotions were too big for my little frame to handle; they seemed to swallow me whole. My emotional state dictated the choices I made. I thought this state was normal. Anxiety was not something that people spoke about.

My sleep was sporadic and without any structure. The impact of this anxiety on my sleep was not positive and created an unfortunate cycle. I never saw the link. I would sleep for hours in the middle of the day to escape feeling, and I would stay up late fretting or partying till the early hours. The next morning, I would lie awake in bed for hours, with zero motivation to get up. I didn't want to face the day.

My bed became a hiding place and sleep an anaesthetic.

By the time I reached my late twenties, I was on a much better path, and I was returning to my true self. I began psychotherapy when my son was very young, and I went every week for a period of two years. Each week I would sit there and wonder why I had come. I was fine. And then I would cry. I cried and wondered if the tears would ever stop. They did.

The crying healed me. The therapy was very hard as I slowly began to unravel what was behind those tears. Therapy is not for the faint-hearted; it requires courage. It was an integral step to the positive mental health I enjoy today. But what truly elevates my mental, emotional and physical well-being is hypnotherapy.

When I was ten years old, my dad sat me on his knee and drew a picture of his heart. He drew his aorta and the three arteries that pump blood into the heart. He then got a pen and coloured in one and a half of the arteries to show that they were blocked. He was 39 years old. He received a triple bypass and had a chance at living again. In order to stay alive, one of the most important changes he needed to make was giving up a heavy smoking habit. My dad is a poet, and his study was right next to my bedroom (I had my own room by then) with a thin partition wall between us. Every night as I slept, my dad listened to hypnosis tapes suggesting that he would never smoke again, and he didn't.

Hypnosis helped to save my father's life and it totally transformed mine. Programming my subconscious with repetitive positive suggestions has brought me home to who I am. My true self is that happy-go-lucky seven-year-old who is not afraid to speak her mind, sleeps like a rock, wakes up early with positive energy, laughs out loud and does her best to make the world a little bit better.

My relationship with sleep has matured over time and I now realise that in order for me to cultivate what I once took for granted at seven years old, it is necessary to emulate my life then. To sleep well, I need to laugh, play, get outside and see the light, to breathe in the sweet air of life, let go and have faith in my innate ability to sleep. At seven years old, I had no real responsibility, which is why these things came more easily.

I hope that at seven, you shared the same freedom to be a child. Still, with each year of life, responsibilities increase, and with them the potential for stress. Viewing responsibility as empowering has helped me tremendously. The different phases of my life have (as for many women) created obstacles to solid sleep – for example, having a baby and entering perimenopause early. Hindsight is worthwhile only if we learn from it and I can see that the biggest challenge of all has been my own mindset – I didn't prioritise effective sleep when I needed it most.

I am now in my late forties, and as I write this book, I am having the best sleep of my life. I thought I was a good sleeper before I started this journey. I can see now that I didn't know what it felt like to be a superb sleeper. One of my best friends, Jane, has an abundance of energy and is the picture of youth and health. Jane has always spoken about her lifelong love affair with sleep. She has a busy life and a huge number of responsibilities that she carries with ease and grace. I admire her greatly. Much of this, she says, is down to her consistently prioritising her sleep. On holidays, she would see me yawn and say, 'You do know, you are not sleeping enough.' 'I AM a good sleeper,' I would insist. 'I just love the early mornings.' She could see the reality, though. I was OK, and I was 'better' than many, but my bar was quite low. Like most people, I didn't know what consistent deep sleep felt like. That is, until I wrote this book and began to experience it night after night.

Jane has always prioritised her sleep above all else, and now I know why. I am so grateful I decided to write this book. Through the small tweaks I have made to my lifestyle and, more important, my mindset, my sleep has reached a new level. I now get to sleep within minutes (it used to take me roughly twenty minutes before I let go). I sleep right through the night, and after years of struggling with my husband's snoring, I rarely hear it now. If I do wake up, I apply the Sleep Well Formula and I almost always get back to sleep immediately. I can sleep on planes, in new places, anywhere.

Like my life, my sleep is not perfect; however, my faith is steadfast. My focus and energy are better than ever before. I continue to take a short nap most days, even though I don't experience the same level of fatigue in the afternoon as I did before. I have a huge respect for sleep and the life it gives me, and I know that this is a relationship I will continue to honour for the rest of my days.

✦ ✦ ✦

Your Sleep Story (So Far!)

THIS EXERCISE IS very revealing. I certainly found it so when I did it myself and it will help you to write your own sleep story.

You need to shed all doubt. It is logical that if sleep once came easily, it can again. So, what is different now? Enter into silence, close your eyes, and take seven full breaths.

Now it is your turn to write your story. You can do so by answering the following questions, which I used as a framework for my own story. You will be amazed at what you learn about yourself when you view your personal history through the lens of sleep. Allow at least 30 minutes to fully explore these questions. This is important, and it will really help bring some powerful insights into your current relationship with sleep.

Take a pen and do this now. Remember, now is the only moment you have.

✦ When was your sleep at its best?

✦ What were you told about your sleep as a baby/toddler?

✦ What did your parents/family tell you about being a good or bad sleeper?

✦ What was your sleep like as a child? Were there any changes in the family? If so, did these affect your sleep?

✦ At what age did your childhood end? In other words, when did you lose the innocence of being a child?

✦ What was your sleep like as a teenager?

✦ What was your sleep like as a young adult?

✦ When was a period of your life when you felt most anxious or stressed?

✦ What is your sleep like now?

You may have some contradictory answers: for example, perhaps the house you lived in was noisy but somehow you slept well, whereas now the slightest creak is likely to disturb you. The most important thing to hold on to is recreating the feeling of trust in your ability to sleep peacefully.

Your story is not finished. I would like you to come back to this at the end of the eight-week programme and again one year from now to answer the following questions:

✦ What is your sleep like now after completing the Sleep Well Programme?

✦ What is your sleep like one year after completing the Sleep Well Programme?

✦ ✦ ✦

Wake Up to the Story You Tell Yourself

AS YOU HAVE seen in both my story and Fionnuala's story on p. 18, we now fully expect to sleep well when we go to bed and, as a result, we do. David Robson is an award-winning science writer specialising in the extremes of the human brain, body and behaviour. I came across his 2022 book *The Expectation Effect* rather serendipitously while writing this one. Robson's robust research in psychology, neuroscience and medicine confirms that your beliefs truly matter not only when it comes to sleep, but in how you perceive pain, lose weight, heal, learn, play sports, the quality of your relationships and how long you will live.

Throughout his book, Robson refers to the brain as 'the prediction machine', and an increasingly large cohort of neuroscientists agree that the brain uses expectations and previous experiences to shape our reality. Anil Seth, professor of cognitive and computational neuroscience and author of *Being You: A New Science of Consciousness*, says, '[T]he brain applies its expectations to our visual reality.'

Your brain works on predictions.

Your brain fills in missing information in your visual perception. When you look at the world around you, your eyes send images to the brain that are often incomplete and unclear. Your brain uses prior knowledge and expectations to fill in the gaps and create a more coherent picture of the world.

For example, if someone you know has recently been the victim of online fraud and you check your account and find a transaction you can't recall making, your brain will jump to the worst-case scenario. You are unconsciously drawing on your friend's unfortunate experience to make sense of the unexplained debit from your account. As you continue to wake up to the automatic patterns of your brain, you begin to see the expectation effect everywhere. Waking up means you are in a position to step back, to allow space and time to see the full picture emerge before jumping to a conclusion. In the example above, even if you *have* been a victim of fraud, you will be in a calmer state of mind to deal with the situation.

The Expectation Effect also explores how your beliefs create your reality on a physical level. As we learned previously, your thoughts have a direct impact on your health and sleep. If you have one 'bad' night's sleep, your brain starts to predict another one. You need to interrupt this pattern, to understand the causes of your disrupted sleep and to gain the perspective that this is a temporary situation and not a permanent problem.

For example, if you convince yourself that you are prone to insomnia, it is likely that you will experience the symptoms of insomnia. In 2018, scientists in Colorado and Oxford recruited 63 people who met the criteria for insomnia disorder. The researchers invited the group of 'bad sleepers' into their sleep laboratory and monitored their brains as they slept. The scientists discovered that, contrary to the participants' negative beliefs, they were getting the recommended minimum of seven hours of sleep.[11]

The following day, when the participants awoke, the scientists gave half the group the good news that their sleep was much better than they had expected it to be. The other half were provided with sham evidence that supported their negative expectations. That evening, all the participants were given a simple cognitive test. The group who had been given positive feedback reported feeling more alert, less fatigued and in a better mood during the day. The group with the fake negative findings showed impaired daytime function, were less focused and felt exhausted. They even showed higher blood pressure, which is a symptom of insomnia. This controlled experiment provides evidence that misperceptions of how you sleep create genuine daytime features of insomnia. The group were not inventing these debilitating symptoms: blood pressure doesn't lie.

Complaining Good Sleepers

PEOPLE WHO BELIEVE their sleep is worse than it is are referred to as 'complaining good sleepers' and the research estimates that 40 per cent of people who have insomnia could belong in this cohort. Robson says, 'This is a lot of suffering to hold on to a needless negative belief about their sleep.' On the reverse, a non-complaining bad sleeper who doesn't feel anxious about their sleep remains miraculously free from the ill effects of poor sleep. The best-case scenario is to be a non-complaining good sleeper. If you believe that you are a bad sleeper, it is time to question this notion.

If you remain unconvinced, another example of how ingrained beliefs shape our reality is the well-known concept of 'baby brain'. This is the time when a woman is pregnant and/or has just given birth and experiences brain fog. Dr Sarah McKay, neuroscientist and author (who shares her sleep story on p. 207), debunks the myth in her latest book, *Baby Brain: The surprising neuroscience of how pregnancy and motherhood sculpt our brains and change our minds (for the better)*. Dr McKay is from New Zealand but now lives in Australia, and the first time she had ever heard of the concept of 'baby brain' was when she went to mother and baby groups in Sydney. The idea didn't exist in her country and therefore it wasn't an issue. Remarkably, studies on the brains of pregnant women show that the boost in oestrogen while we are pregnant actually enhances cognition. Dr McKay says, 'It is definitely not a hormonal thing but a lack of sleep that makes it tough. We tend to find the closest hook to hang our hat on and then blame that. Once we start to look for a reason to feel forgetful or tired or foggy, we go, "Well, it's 'the baby brain'", or if you are over sixty, "it must be Alzheimer's".[12] Hormones, like genetics, can get a bad rap and strip you of a sense of agency over your own health and well-being.

✦ ✦ ✦

Keep the Faith, No Matter What Challenges You Face

AS YOU GO through phases of your life, you will inevitably have different challenges that affect your sleep. Looking at your sleeping habits within the context of your circumstances is essential. It is unfair on yourself to expect to sleep without interruption if you have a new baby or are going through cancer treatment, suffering grief, or caring for an elderly parent during the night. Sleep challenges depending on your phase in life are valid concerns and provide obstacles to your sleep, for example, menopausal hot sweats, chronic pain or a sleep disorder such as insomnia. Rest assured, we will examine the main challenges to sleep in Week Five: Embrace the Challenges.

No matter what subjective sleep challenges you currently face, your personal sleep story, your childhood and cultural conditioning have shaped your brain to make predictions about your ability to sleep. For example, 'I never sleep on a plane' or 'I always have a bad night's sleep before a presentation.' Each of these thoughts creates the very thing you don't wish to manifest. It is time to turn these pessimistic predictions into positive expectations such as 'I sleep easily on a plane' and 'I sleep deeply before a presentation.'

The Sleep Well Formula (Breathe + Imagine + Experience = Faith) must apply no matter what subjective challenges you face now.

It is crucial you do not define yourself by a period in your life when you experienced disrupted sleep. Many people never doubt their ability to sleep until they have a life-changing experience, such as a traumatic event, a stressful job, having a baby, losing a loved one, financial issues, perimenopause or becoming ill. Once their rhythm is broken, they continue to react to a threat that has long since been removed.

No matter how poor your sleep currently is, you will find that you are still asleep for more time than you are awake during the night.

Even if you have a chronic health condition, such as ongoing pain, diabetes or asthma, which can all impinge upon sleep, you will still find you have more hours of slumber than wakefulness. If you find yourself thinking, 'I am not sure if I was asleep at all,' after a fitful night in bed, it is likely you were. You are simply hypervigilant during the lighter phases of sleep, and so the perception of being awake seems real. In Week Four, I will explain the five different phases of sleep and the benefits of each phase. For now, it is important to know that we all enter into light phases of sleep every night. Those who are aware of this lighter phase will be in a higher state of arousal and break through to a more wakeful state. Accepting the fact that you are in a lighter phase of sleep, that this is natural, and no longer seeing it as a problem means that you will drift back to sleep more quickly.

When you remove the pressure to have eight hours straight of perfect sleep, you will find that more often than not this is what you get. The eight habits in the Sleep Well Programme offer scientific and practical protocols that *will* help you to sleep better. You can meticulously implement each one, but if your mindset is stuck in a negative belief that 'you can't sleep well' then you will continue to struggle. The best mattress in the world, a night nurse to feed your babies, hormone replacement therapy, nothing will change your ability to sleep well if you do not have faith that you can.

Consider other unhelpful beliefs that you may have once had and have now let go of. For example, perhaps you once believed you could never become a vegetarian, stop smoking, take financial control of your life or sustain an exercise routine. Find a positive habit that you have already cultivated in your life and feel your confidence grow.

✦ ✦ ✦

The Negative Feedback Loop

TODAY IS THE day you become a non-complaining good sleeper. Do you currently hear yourself saying any of the following?

✦ 'I'm a bad sleeper.'

✦ 'I'm a light sleeper.'

✦ 'I have trouble falling asleep.'

✦ 'I struggle with staying asleep throughout the night.'

✦ 'I toss and turn all night.'

- ✦ 'I wake up frequently during the night.'

- ✦ 'I suffer from insomnia.'

- ✦ 'I never sleep through the night.'

- ✦ 'I feel tired and groggy in the mornings.'

- ✦ 'Sleep is elusive to me.'

- ✦ 'I have trouble getting my beauty sleep.'

- ✦ 'I'm always wide awake when I should be sleeping.'

- ✦ 'My mind just races when I go to bed.'

- ✦ 'I have trouble shutting off my brain at night.'

- ✦ 'I've always been a poor sleeper.'

- ✦ 'I'm a chronic insomniac.'

- ✦ 'I'm a zombie in the mornings.'

- ✦ 'I'm constantly exhausted.'

If you answered 'Yes' to any of the above, it is time to change the programme, both in what you say and how you think about sleep. This is going to take practice, but it is an essential step to your liberation. As long as you continue to affirm any of the above, no change is possible. Remember to practise this not only with the thoughts in your mind but also with what you say out loud to other people.

Each time you complain about your sleep not being good enough, you are creating a negative feedback loop. The people in your life expect you to sleep badly and your 'bad sleep' becomes a point of conversation. They will show you empathy and concern, but rather than helping you, they will keep you stuck in an identity you no longer wish to hold.

With your head up high, it is time to say:

+ 'I am a good sleeper.'

+ 'I sleep through anything.'

+ 'I sleep soundly throughout the night and wake up refreshed.'

+ 'I have peaceful and uninterrupted nights of sleep.'

+ 'I'm a deep sleeper; once I'm out, I'm out!'

+ 'I'm out like a light as soon as my head hits the pillow.'

+ 'I enjoy a consistently good night's sleep.'

+ 'I experience deep, rejuvenating sleep every night.'

+ 'I have developed healthy sleep patterns that promote optimal rest.'

+ 'My nights are peaceful, and my sleep is uninterrupted.'

+ 'I wake up feeling refreshed and energised each morning.'

+ 'I wake up gently and ease myself into the day.'

+ 'I love my sleep.'

+ 'I look forward to bedtime.'

I know this may sound like a stretch, yet, with time, these aspirations become your lived experience. As your sleep is in a transitional stage, it is best to simply state that you are on a sleep journey and are making positive changes.

The people in your life will most likely be bewildered; they may even question your sanity. When you change a behaviour, even for the positive, it can cause ripples amongst the people in your life. Explain that you are going through a period of transition and ask them for their patience. Over time, your improved sleep will encourage them to improve their own relationship to it. You become a force of positive change for the people you love.

As you relinquish the labels you have given yourself regarding your ability to sleep, it is also important to let go of comparing your sleep to that of others or getting competitive about it.

Sleep is not a competition.

It seems strange that we feel envy when we think that someone else has better or more sleep than us, but we do. Consider the sleep wars that can exist between new parents, or siblings who are minding elderly parents. Frustration can build into resentment and those negative feelings create another block to quality sleep or, indeed, an arrow to fire at yourself.

✦ ✦ ✦

An Empowering Parable to Sleep and to Live By

IN PSYCHOLOGY, WE have primary and secondary emotional responses, but long before these terms were invented, the Buddha talked about our emotional reactions in terms of arrows.

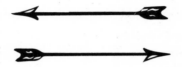

In this image, the first arrow represents a difficulty in your life or indeed in your sleep and the second is your response. For example:

✦ The first arrow is a chronic health issue that wakes you up. This is not something you have chosen or have control over.

✦ The second arrow is how you react when you are woken up – and this you do have agency over.

In Buddhism, they say, 'Pain is inevitable, suffering is optional.' Pain is part of being human: to avoid suffering you need to accept pain, and resistance only adds to it.

The steps to do this are the following and they can be used in any challenging situation you have with sleep or indeed in life.

- Recognise when the first arrow hits. Feel the pain and note what you are experiencing in your body. Pain can be emotional also.

- Accept the pain/anxiety without the impulse to wish it was not there. You accept the moment as it is.

- Breathe into the discomfort while allowing it to be there. It will slowly ease as you breathe into it.

- Allow any thoughts and feelings to be there – you do not need to fix the situation or identify with it. It will pass and you will get back to sleep.

- Cultivate a sense of self-compassion, admitting to yourself that this is not easy, but you are managing the situation.

You can practise these steps for any issue that is out of your control in your life while you are in bed or fully awake.

Compassion will triumph over frustration. Acceptance of your challenges will set you free to open the door to sleep night after night.

✦ ✦ ✦

Build Your Sleep Well Habits

PLEASE CONTINUE TO practise Habit One – 'Go to sleep and wake up at roughly the same time each day'. I'm sure it is not perfect, and nor do we want it to be. The idea is *roughly* the same time. If you get completely out of the routine, just start again the next day.

It is now time to introduce the very soothing and essential next habit. Remember that you can stack your habits together to create cues in your neural circuitry to help take the pressure off.

HABIT TWO

Create a 'Blissful Hour' 60-Minute Bedtime Routine

To experience peace does not mean that your life is always blissful. It means that you are capable of tapping into a blissful state of mind amidst the normal chaos of a hectic life.

JILL BOLTE TAYLOR,

NEUROSCIENTIST AND AUTHOR

OF MY STROKE OF INSIGHT

DON'T MISTAKE 'SLEEP time' for 'bedtime'. They are two different things. Bedtime is when you commence the journey to sleep. In the same way that you need time to get ready in the morning before your day begins, you also need time to unwind for sleep.

Start this ritual 60 minutes before you want to be asleep. Creating your very own hour of bliss to unwind your mind means that by the time you want to be asleep, your body and mind are ready. The blissful hour becomes a habit you genuinely look forward to. You learn to relish the time to disconnect from the outside world and enter into a deeper connection with yourself. The gentle unwinding process encourages you to let go of roles, responsibilities, the future and the past and truly nourish yourself. When your nervous system is relaxed going to sleep, you will automatically feel safe, which is, as you know, essential for getting to sleep and staying asleep.

Create the routine that suits you best. It should consist of a variety of low-stress activities that are designed to activate the parasympathetic (rest and digest) nervous system and help you to feel relaxed and at ease. The parasympathetic system decreases your heart rate, which helps the body to relax and restore energy. This restful state creates homeostasis (balance in your system) and a low level of arousal that signals to the body it is safe to go to sleep. Your blissful hour is time to consciously slow down your breathing. As you brush your teeth and undress, begin to breathe more deeply and serenely as this will send the signal that sleep is imminent.

Some ideas to include in your blissful hour are:

✦ Guided or silent meditation

✦ Reading fiction or poetry

✦ Taking a hot bath or shower

✦ Aromatherapy

✦ Drinking chamomile/lavender/night-time tea

✦ Listening to soothing music or nature sounds

✦ Practising breathing rituals, such as the cyclic sigh, which you will learn in Week Three.

- ✦ Gentle yoga such as restorative or yin

- ✦ Making love or sexual self-pleasuring

- ✦ Journaling – see below for some sleep time journaling suggestions.

Journaling

I have kept a diary since I was 12 years old, and it is a companion that is always there for me. Sometimes I write a lot, sometimes a little. There are two types of journaling. The first is free-style and you allow whatever comes into your mind to be released onto the page. This is very therapeutic and can be especially helpful when you need to make sense of your emotional landscape. Writing your stream of consciousness helps you to make connections that can simply spin around in the brain if they are left to their own devices.

Research shows that expressive writing helps the brain to 'cool down' when it has entered a state of anxiety. Hans Schroder, the lead researcher on a study conducted at Michigan State University, said, 'Worrying takes up cognitive resources; it's kind of like people who struggle with worry are constantly multitasking – they are doing one task and trying to monitor and suppress their worries at the same time. Our findings show that if you get these worries out of your head through expressive writing, those cognitive resources are freed up to work toward the task you're completing, and you become more efficient.'[13]

Question negative thoughts. Don't let them spin around in your mind – get them out and onto the page.

Free-style Journaling

Take out the mental garbage. First thing in the morning or last thing at night, allow your pen to flow as you literally clear out the thoughts that have been spinning around. You feel so much better when you do this as there is no need to carry them with you all day or night!

Reflective Journaling

The second type of journaling is reflective journaling, in which you use prompts with the intention to write about something specific, for example gratitude. In the field of positive psychology, there has been a lot of research into the benefits of keeping a gratitude journal. Leading researchers in the field Robert Emmons and Michael McCullough have found that keeping a daily gratitude journal improves the quality of our sleep, brings us closer to others, creates more happiness and even reduces physical pain.[14]

I have given you some of these prompts throughout the book and they are effective for discovering more about yourself. The prompts below are designed to calm your mind, soothe your soul and prepare you for a peaceful night's sleep.

The following bedtime journaling routine is one that I personally follow. You can choose one or all of the prompts – it totally depends on what works for you.

Gratitude for the Good

Find the gold in your day. Be specific: it can be small moments of presence and stillness that you recall, such as gazing at a flower or laughing with a friend. Look for the good in your day, and you will find it. I recommend finding three things.

Gratitude for the Challenges

What obstacles did you overcome in your day? We don't often show gratitude for the difficulties in our lives, yet this is where we learn most about ourselves. Find at least one example: it could be that you were irritated with your mother, but mindfully let it go, or you stayed focused to meet a deadline.

Emotional Intention for Tomorrow

Write down how you wish to be and to feel the next day. Visualise the day you have planned and see yourself operate from this chosen emotional state. You can also journal what goals you would like to accomplish (not with pressure but with compassion). Again, be specific. This practice is very powerful because as you sleep your subconscious will soak in your intentions and help them to become a reality.

Three Questions to Ask Yourself

✦ What do I need to let go of?

✦ What do I need to embrace?

✦ How can I make the world a better place tomorrow?

Boundaries

Create boundaries around your blissful hour with the people you love. Be clear on this before you begin your 60 minutes to unwind, especially if you have children or teenagers. Ask them if there is anything they need to say, to speak now or hold their silence until the morning. If you do not have clear boundaries, you will be constantly interrupted.

Also, explain to family and friends that you won't be available unless it is an emergency. It sounds selfish. It isn't. Your best-slept self will be fully able to help others when you are refreshed and emotionally regulated.

Explain to your partner, if you have one, that this hour is not the time to discuss anything stressful or even exciting. You want to empty your mind, not fill it. Invite your family to be part of this blissful hour (as long as they respect the rituals). You can unwind together, and it is a precious time to bond through peace.

Ben Nemtin, the bestselling author of *What Do You Want To Do Before You Die?*, practises the following 'Rose' bedtime ritual with his family. They come together and share what was 'the bud' of their day, something that is growing within; what was the thorn, a challenge they faced; and what was the rose, the part of their day they are most grateful for. This is also a lovely exercise to do solo.

What this Looks Like for Me
I often meditate before bed for 15 minutes with the scent of lavender incense and a cup of chamomile tea. Sometimes I have a hot shower or bath, especially if I have a big event the next day or I am travelling. I journal and then read a good novel. When I break my routine for social or travel reasons and I am in bed later than normal, I forgo these practices, but will always, always read before sleep.

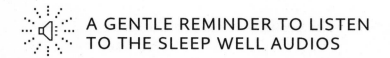

A GENTLE REMINDER TO LISTEN TO THE SLEEP WELL AUDIOS

You can access these audios for FREE with the passcode ISLEEPWELL on www.thepositivehabit.com.

Please remember to listen to the instructions for listening to guarantee maximum benefits.

MORNING MEDITATION

Please listen each morning to 'Start Your Day in Stillness – Intention-Setting Morning Meditation' to slow down your thoughts, before the day commences.

AFTERNOON OR EVENING REST RITUAL

Please listen to 'Seven-Minute Rest Ritual' each afternoon and/or evening.

NIGHT-TIME HYPNOTHERAPY – WEEK TWO: HABIT TWO

This is the most important track to listen to. Each week there are new subconscious suggestions to help to reinforce the corresponding weekly habit and the following key insights.

To Get Back to Sleep if You Wake Up

YOU CAN LISTEN to your night-time audio again, if necessary, but with time you will not need to do this. The Sleep Well Formula (Breathe + Imagine + Experience = Faith) which you are learning on a subconscious level every time you listen to your weekly audios will become automatic. Please also listen to the '4, 7, 8 Breathing' audio and train yourself to do this in the middle of the night should you awaken.

THE GOLDEN KEY INSIGHTS FROM WEEK TWO: YOUR SLEEP STORY

- ✦ There is a scientific door to sleep that you can open each night when you provide a conducive environment and positive mindset – all of which you are implementing in this book.

- ✦ In order to go to sleep you need to feel safe physically, mentally and emotionally. When you feel safe, you are in a position to welcome sleep.

- ✦ Having written your own sleep story, you are learning to change the narrative of what no longer serves you. The thoughts in your voice matter and positive affirmations such as 'I am a good sleeper' and 'I experience deep, rejuvenating sleep every night' will change the narrative.

- ✦ Expectations can have a placebo or nocebo effect on your ability to sleep well.

- ✦ You will enter lighter phases of sleep, and accepting these moments of semi-consciousness ensures that you will return to a deeper sleep more quickly.

- ✦ Your faith in your innate ability to sleep well is at the heart of your sleep success.

- ✦ Habit Two is 'Create a "blissful hour" 60-minute bedtime routine'.

To maximise the benefits of this programme, I encourage you not to begin reading Week Three until you have listened to the 'Week Two: Habit Two' night-time audio for a minimum of seven nights in total.

✦ ✦ ✦

Keep going – you are doing really well. I have faith in you. Please remember to acknowledge all progress with your habits and mindset, no matter how big or small.

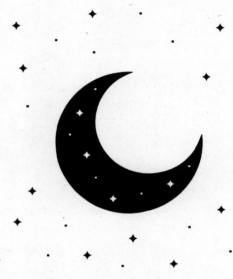

YOUR WAKING SELF

Whatever you impress upon your subconscious mind, the latter will move heaven and earth to bring it to pass. You must therefore impress it with right ideas and constructive thoughts.

WILLIAM JAMES (1842–1910)

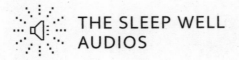

THE SLEEP WELL AUDIOS

All audios are available to download on www.thepositivehabit.com with the password ISLEEPWELL.

✦ Tonight, please start listening to 'Week Three: Habit Three' of the Sleep Well audios. Please listen to this audio for a minimum of seven nights. Please do not skip ahead to Week Four until you have listened for a full seven days.

✦ Please also continue to listen to your morning meditation and your rest ritual tracks each day.

✦ ✦ ✦

Measure Your Sleep

BEFORE YOU BEGIN Week Three of the Sleep Well Programme, please take a moment to rate your sleep. On a scale of 0 to 10, how well have you slept in the last week? (0 is 'terribly' and 10 is 'very well'.) Please use the image on the opposite page to mark where you feel you are on this scale.

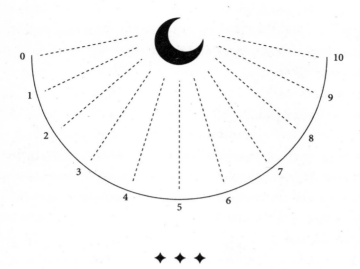

✦ ✦ ✦

Welcome to Week Three

I HOPE YOU have been enjoying your blissful hour habit; many people create a morning routine but neglect to cultivate a night-time one. It makes sense to bookend our days with presence. Wherever you are on your sleep journey, embrace it and remember that patience is one of the strengths you are building. This week, you will examine your subconscious mind in its waking state and learn how essential it is to move from unconscious, conditioned and often maladaptive thought patterns to conscious, unconditioned and adaptive ones. For example, moving from an unconscious bias of not feeling worthy to one of valuing yourself. You will harness the power of your subconscious mind to know the difference between constructive imagination and catastrophising – for example, imagining a positive outcome for a health diagnosis as opposed to suspecting the worst-case scenario. You will liberate yourself from automatic negative thoughts that hijack your nervous system and keep you awake at night and asleep during the day. Rest assured, the positive suggestions included in the Sleep Well hypnotherapy audios are impressing the 'right ideas' and 'constructive thoughts' into your subconscious mind as you sleep.

You will learn about the collective awakening to valuing our sleep as the cornerstone of health. I am also excited to share with you the sleep story of yogi and assistant professor of medicine at Harvard Medical School Sat Bir Singh Khalsa. Sat Bir has spent many years researching various states of consciousness, including sleep and the higher level of consciousness that is induced by yoga and meditation.

✦ ✦ ✦

Visiting Your Subconscious

WHY DO YOU need to visit your subconscious in its waking state? The reason is that a lack of self-knowledge surrounding your own emotional history and subconscious belief systems means that you will unintentionally repeat mistakes from the past. This default to habits both behavioural and emotional can be very dysfunctional. For example, if as a child you wanted to be seen as a good girl or boy and did all you could to please your parents, you could find yourself many years later working into the late hours of the night, forgoing sleep to gain the approval of your boss. You still want to be that 'good boy or girl'. You are simply not aware of what is driving your behaviour.

Once you understand the roots of your behaviour, you are in a position to change it.

It takes eight hours to change your life night after night. Repetition is a prerequisite to carving new pathways into the neural structure of your brain. Imagine you show a child love just once or even a handful of times in their entire life. Do you think they will feel safe with you? Safe enough to sleep in your arms? Most likely not. Your subconscious self is that child and needs to hear the message that it is loved time and time again to feel secure and to fall asleep.

My voice in your night-time audios is your loving guardian, bringing you home to that 'unwounded space' within you, where sleep comes effortlessly.

As you listen, your mind will invariably wander. Each time it does, simply return your focus to my voice to access your subconscious sweet spot where sustainable change happens.

To get to know your subconscious self, you need to visit it when it is at home, both in its waking and its sleeping state. During the day, when you drift into automatic mode, your subconscious will dictate your emotions, habits and behaviours if you are not aware of it. At night, your subconscious is waiting patiently in the wings for your conscious mind to go offline. It is like an understudy in a play, hoping the lead actor will give them a chance to show the world their true talent.

The Awake Subconscious Self

WHEN YOU ARE awake and idle, for example waiting for someone or lying in bed, your mind will inevitably wander. In this state, the default mode network (DMN) is activated; the DMN is located in various regions of the brain including the prefrontal cortex and medial temporal lobe. These regions are often involved in tasks related to self-referential thinking and pondering on how other people perceive us. This is why you might find yourself in bed ruminating on what you said or didn't say at a meeting/social occasion. You are not present here and now; instead you are mentally time-travelling. Your mind will project you into the future and pull you into the past. (This is 'psychological time' at work, which is a concept we will explore more in Week Six: Presence.) When you get into bed at night, if you haven't taken the necessary time to unwind your mind it will slip into this default state and it will keep you awake. This is why last week's habit (creating a 'blissful hour' 60-minute bedtime routine) is so important.

There is growing evidence that the DMN is also active during repetitive and familiar tasks when you are busy.[15] For example, you may be physically driving on a familiar route, but your mind has wandered off to a holiday you are looking forward to or ruminating on a difficult meeting you had yesterday at work. Your body is in one place – the now (the car) – and your mind is somewhere else – the future (the holiday) or the past (the meeting) – and yet somehow you arrive safely. You are on autopilot and your subconscious is driving the car for you.

Mind-wandering has its advantages. In the example above, the benefit is clear: you arrive alive and, in addition, your brain is free to wander. As the mind meanders, solutions to problems can emerge. Have you ever had one of those 'Aha' moments when you least expected it? Perhaps you have been worrying endlessly about an issue and then, while you are on a walk or staring out your window, it becomes crystal clear what you need to do.

Your subconscious mind already had the answer; it simply required the freedom to roam and to present it to you.

A marvellous benefit of the DMN is the creation of innovative ideas and masterful works of creativity. When the mind wanders, the brain is free to make associations between various pieces of information without any pressure. For example, it is said that Einstein came up with his groundbreaking theory of relativity while daydreaming about riding a beam of light. J.K. Rowling invented Harry Potter while waiting for a delayed train.

Allowing your mind to wander is a necessary and highly positive thing to do – on occasion. It is the amount of time spent wandering that causes difficulties. Being on automatic pilot for most of your life disconnects you from presence, and from those you love. You are more caught up with the fantasy in your mind than the reality of the moment. In other words, you are not aware of your external surroundings, including the people you are with. If you have ever had the feeling of being spaced out at a meeting or while chatting to a friend, and struggled to catch up with the conversation, you will know what I am referring to. In addition, the 'awake subconscious' has a magnetic pull that takes you away from calmness and gives your ego full reign. For example, the person who is ruminating while driving will be quick to anger at the car that pulls out suddenly in front of them, as opposed to the more mindful driver who remains tranquil and hence has a faster response mechanism.

Making Conscious Choices

WHEN YOU BECOME lost in thought it is easy to fall into negative and repetitive cycles. These thoughts spin around in a circle that never ends. If you remain oblivious to the origin of these thoughts, the subconscious memory that causes them to be so intense means you will simply fall into the same trap time and time again.

The well-known poem by Portia Nelson 'Autobiography in Five Short Chapters' depicts this message so poignantly. She writes her life in five chapters. In the first chapter, she walks down a street and sees a deep hole on the footpath. She falls in and feels hopeless and it takes her a long time to get out. In the second chapter, she walks down the same street and doesn't see the hole. She falls in and claims it is not her fault, she can't believe she is back there, and again it takes an age to get out of it. In the third chapter, she walks down the same street, she sees the hole and still falls in. It has become a habit, but she takes responsibility for it and climbs out quickly. In the fourth chapter, she walks down the same street, sees the hole and walks around it. In the fifth, very short, chapter she simply walks down another street.

Consider what holes you keep falling into. Each of us has our 'metaphorical holes', a repeated negative narrative that we tell ourselves about a situation or relationship in our lives. Often, we blame others or society for the situation. The only way to walk down a different street is to become aware – to pull yourself out of subconscious habits into conscious choices.

The following two daytime practices will help you do this. They are:

✦ Formal meditation

✦ Informal 'on the go' mindfulness

FORMAL MEDITATION

There is a Zen proverb that says, 'If you don't have time to meditate for an hour every day, you should meditate for two hours.' Perhaps you are a seasoned meditator or perhaps you feel that it sounds like too much hard work, and you don't have the time or maybe even the interest. Either way, the science shows a sitting meditation of just five minutes a day will help you to understand the inner workings of your automatic thoughts.

There are many different types of meditation, from transcendental (which uses a mantra) to specific guided ones that can induce feelings of calmness and relaxation. For the purpose of recognising subconscious thought patterns and narratives, an anchor-based breath mindfulness method is best.

In a formal practice, you sit in an upright position, close your eyes or lower your gaze and focus your mind on your inhale and exhale. You will notice just how quickly your internal voice begins to chatter. Meditation is the practice of refocusing your attention each time it wanders. It is this process of watching your mind that sets you free. As you are already listening to the 'Start Your Day in Stillness – Intention-Setting Morning Meditation', you will be, I hope, seeing some of the benefits of slowing down your mind and observing your thoughts.

You will begin to see patterns and, most important, realise that you are not the voice in your mind but the presence that observes it.

For example, if you cut your finger, you can observe the cut and the blood that pours; you can say to yourself, 'This cut is sore, it is hurting me.' You can do the same thing with your thoughts. This is a subtle process and requires patience. Your thoughts have the power to hurt or heal you. With practice, you will begin to see closely the nature of your thoughts and the harmful patterns that emerge time and time again.

Sitting with yourself in silence and stillness is an act of love. You are not trying to run away or distract yourself from yourself. A formal meditation practice interrupts the automatic pilot pattern. You become aware of your thoughts, feelings and beliefs so that you make conscious choices. You begin to understand why you behave the way you do.

A recent randomised trial carried out in 2022 on 108 participants, led by Professor Andrew Huberman and Dr Dan Spiegel at Stanford University, indicated that just five minutes of breath-based meditation a day is sufficient to reduce anxiety and improve your mood.[16] Each of the volunteers was given stress reduction exercises to practise for five minutes a day for four weeks. They were asked to keep a stress journal and to observe their progress. The results showed that all of the interventions helped, but those who used breathing exercises had calmer nervous systems. Within this cohort, those who were given the following exercise, known as the cyclic sigh, had lower heart rates, less tension and better focus.

+ Breathe in through your nose, pause, and then take a second short inhale. The first inhale is longer than the second, but the second inhale is equally important to ensure your lungs fill to their full capacity.

+ Breathe out a very elongated sigh through your mouth.

+ Do this for five minutes and then notice how you feel compared to before you started.

Three rounds are enough to feel more relaxed and help to induce sleep. Dr Spiegel refers to this technique as mental kinaesthetics. You know how to breathe, yet in order to utilise the full power of the breath, you need to hone the art.

You are becoming a proactive agent in calming your own nervous system.

INFORMAL 'ON THE GO' MINDFULNESS

Mindfulness on the go is when you apply the same principle of observation that you have in your formal meditation practice to your everyday life. The meditation bell doesn't stop ringing. Bringing the quality of presence you have cultivated in your formal practice (no matter how short) to daily life is the ultimate liberation. In my first book, *The Positive Habit*, I explored the triggers that can pull you from presence and into reactivity. Common triggers are those things outside your control: other people, situations and changes to plans. To recognise these triggers, and there are many, watch yourself as though you are observing a child you love.

Develop an infinite compassionate curiosity towards yourself. Become fascinated with why you behave the way you do, the nature of your thoughts, the sensations of your emotions within your body, how you interact with the people you love, your colleagues, and your neighbours, and notice how you change when you are in the company of different people – how does your voice change, the language you use, with whom do you present your best self and why? Who sees you at your most impatient? Again, why? Where do you carry tension in your body? When and where does it stiffen? When and where does it relax? How do you feel after a good night's sleep as opposed to a restless one?

Can you see the connection between your best self and your best-slept self?

Through this gentle yet consistent awareness, you witness emotional patterns emerging, and by noticing them you start to interrupt them. A key component of mindfulness is about clearing and cleansing internal emotional disturbances as they arise. This cleansing process ensures you sleep well. You choose to let go of emotional pain rather than letting it accumulate and build up over the course of the day – or indeed a lifetime.

THE ARC MINDFULNESS TOOL
My three-step mindfulness tool ARC provides a highly practical and powerful way to do this in real time. It only takes a few moments once you become skilled at it. You metaphorically walk under an arc to transform fear into love, overwhelm into calmness, and anger into positive action.

Over time, ARC becomes a subconscious and spontaneous response that allows you to sleep peacefully and create harmony with others.

Acceptance

The first step is A for 'Acceptance'. Acceptance is the beginning of a transformation. Change is impossible if you remain in denial, and this applies to yourself, other people, events and circumstances. For example, if you make a mistake, accepting it allows you to learn from it; denying it means that you repeat it. If you are in a toxic relationship and you can't accept that your partner is emotionally abusive and narcissistic, you remain at their mercy and become a victim. For most people, this initial step is often the hardest part.

> The curious paradox is that when I accept myself, just as I am, then I can change.
>
> CARL ROGERS

Resistance, suppression and distraction are the most common forms of trying to cope with situations, people and emotions that cause us suffering. These coping mechanisms are illusory and help you to survive during the day, but when you go to bed at night the same intense thoughts and emotions you suppressed or denied come tumbling in. To go beyond survival, you need to go into those dark spaces when you are wide awake.

One client told me, 'I am so scared to go there, to that place where I feel too much. If I do, I am afraid I won't come back.' The opposite is true. You do come back, renewed, strong and vibrant. Remember, in my personal sleep story, I cried myself to emotional freedom through weekly therapy sessions. Feeling the full range of human emotions enriches your life. From joy to sorrow, each one is a gift. It is understandable why many people struggle to give their emotions free rein. They fear that they will be out of control and unable to function. There is a balance between suppression and being at the mercy of emotion and it is to observe whatever arises with love.

The act of acceptance is instantly soothing. Emotions soften spontaneously.

Try this now. Consider a small issue you have in your life, such as a person you love who is rude to you, or a colleague at work who is asking too much of you. Can you, just now, accept this person, this situation and the frustration it brings, and see what happens in your body? You should notice a small shift, a softening inside as you let go of resistance. (Remember that this is just the first step!)

Unprocessed emotion and chronic stress cause inflammation in the body. As soon as you feel the discomfort of a difficult emotion in your body, accept it. Allow it to move through your body. Consider your body as a river. Just like a river, it is always changing. If you block the flow of your emotions, you will stagnate. Many people describe feeling 'stuck' and this is often because they remain disconnected from their emotions.

Acceptance and commitment therapy (ACT) was founded by psychologist, professor and author Stephen Hayes. ACT is a form of psychotherapy that encourages the client to develop what Hayes refers to as 'psychological flexibility'. This is the ability to remain in the present moment when difficult thoughts, feelings, memories and bodily sensations arise. In doing so, you are able to stay connected to your values and align your actions to meet them.

For example, you feel upset when you indirectly find out your mother is ill and she hadn't told you. You value honesty and caring for those you love. Accepting the situation means that you can explain to her that you would prefer to know in the future so that you can be there to help. Getting frustrated with her or denying her illness will only cause more stress.

Accepting pain, bearing the unbearable and sitting with uncomfortable emotions are paramount to sleeping peacefully.

A 2020 meta-analysis study published in the *Journal of Contextual Behavioral Science* examined 12,477 participants on the efficacy of applying ACT therapy. The results showed that ACT helped to alleviate all the conditions they looked at, including anxiety, depression, substance use and chronic pain.[17]

If you feel anxious, you feel anxious. Don't fight it. Accepting reality, no matter how hard it is, is the first and most critical step to living and sleeping in peace.

Release

The second step of the ARC mindfulness tool is R for 'Release'. Once you have accepted a situation, you are in a position to let it go. This takes practice and also depends on the scale of what it is you wish to release. Perhaps it is a feeling of disappointment in a loved one, or it is more severe, like the pain of grief.

> Sometimes you don't realise the weight of something you have been carrying until you feel the weight of its release.
>
> ANONYMOUS

You will know when the time is right to move forward. The more minor the incident, the quicker you can release.

Recall the idea of radical surrendering from Week Two. Going to and staying asleep is essentially the art of letting go. You hand over control from the conscious mind to the subconscious. A liberated mind and open heart do not cling to ideas, thoughts or personal perspectives of how the world must be.

If you are a person who believes that you are good at letting things go, only for them to resurface later on, you are not alone. For example, your partner was irritable with you in the morning, and you chose not to react, but later that day, you are tired and you snap at them in unconscious retaliation. Or in the middle of an argument, you hear yourself say, 'And another thing ...', recounting a situation from the past that you had 'let go'.

Releasing is about cleansing and clearing each day.

Choosing not to let stress accumulate means there is no tidal wave of emotion waiting for you when you switch the light off at night.

It is imperative to release emotions from where they are stored in the body. The two most powerful ways to release are:

Tears
When you feel tears burning at the edge of your eyes, let them flow. Many people try to push tears down as they equate crying with a sign of weakness. This blockage can feel like a golf ball has got stuck in their throat. The fear of being seen to cry is common. Parents often hide tears from their children, not wanting to upset them; still, children know when something is wrong. They feel it. Seeing a parent cry teaches the child that emotion is human, and tears are transformative, not something to be ashamed of. Clearly, this is done within the context of what is appropriate to share with a child and not as a method to offload onto them. Men and fathers in particular can struggle with this. Patriarchal conditioning teaches us that men who cry are feeble. However, authentic tears cannot be forced or manufactured. Trust that if

you have tears to cry, they will come – and when they do, greet them with joy. Please don't hold back.

Crying is nature's way of allowing emotions to literally flow like a river through your system, so you are cleansed and refreshed. From an evolutionary perspective, emotional tears serve two main purposes. First, they are a powerful way to self-soothe as when you cry you activate your parasympathetic (rest and digest) nervous system.[18] Second, they evolved to elicit empathy from others and help you to form close bonds.[19] Consider the close relationships in your life: is there a degree of shared vulnerability that allows you to feel safe?

Ever wonder why you feel so much better and lighter after a good cry? Crying releases oxytocin and feel-good hormones which elevate your mood, so much so that laughter often follows tears. Children are experts at this as they dance from despair to elation within moments. If you remain unconvinced of the emotional benefits of crying, on a physical level it is said that tears help to kill bacteria and keep the eyes clean by releasing a fluid called lysozyme that contains powerful antimicrobial properties.[20]

When you make space in your life for tears, whether you cry in your therapist's room, with a friend, or on your own, the tears become less necessary and less frequent. This also prevents you from pushing back tears when it is not appropriate to be vulnerable. The more you allow yourself to feel upset, the less upset you feel.

Remember that crying is an act of courage.

Create a safe space and give yourself permission to cry when you feel it and observe how soundly you sleep afterwards.

Shake It Off

All mammals shake. Watch a dog and you will see they do it often: any time they have been still for a period of time, asleep or resting, they rise, stretch and shake. *Why Zebras Don't Get Ulcers* is a best-selling book by neurobiologist Robert Sapolsky. The title says it all: zebras and other animals know how to dissipate stress as it arises. They shake it off and get back to living in the moment. The physical release is a way of transitioning from one state to another. Choosing to shake off stress as soon as you begin to feel it is a very adaptive way of releasing old, stagnant and negative energy and tension from your body.

When you shake with fear this is called a neurogenic tremor, and it is a primal response to threat. Take the fear of public speaking or the experience of a traumatic shock: many people will start to automatically shake. These tremors are part of your survival mechanism: they naturally help to reduce overactivity in the body's complex neuroendocrine system, which regulates your fear response, your feelings and where you store energy.

This adaptive response has been suppressed in humankind through cultural conditioning, as shaking is seen as something to stop, not to encourage. Shaking is seen as a sign of weakness, like tears; however, both of these primitive responses are designed to restore balance to your nervous system. You need to harness the healing power of shaking as part of your commitment to sleep peacefully.

Like meditation, shaking can be done formally and informally, depending on your environment. For example, in a work meeting, you might simply shake your hands out under a table to release the frustration you feel. A walk at lunchtime to shake off the stress is also very beneficial. Once you have released, you are ready to progress to the third and best step of the ARC method.

Compassion

All compassion must commence with self-compassion, which is a subtle art, and again it does not come easily for most people.

> Treat yourself as you would a good friend.
>
> Dr Kristin Neff

However, take solace and remember you have been through the most challenging part of the ARC method: acceptance. You may struggle with self-compassion if you were not taught as a child to show yourself kindness. Self-love was seen as selfish. It is of course imperative that we care for others – but this is impossible unless you have the energy to do this from a fullness within.

To help you with this, do this short reflective exercise. I have given you some examples based on a person in my life.

Choose a friend or family member who accepts you as you are.

Orla, my sister.

What three qualities do you admire most in them?

Humour, genuine empathy, she's always there for me.

What would it be like to apply the same three same qualities to yourself when you feel upset?

It feels liberating and very reassuring to know I can rely on myself to self-soothe and to accept myself as I am.

Compassion is love in action.

Self-compassion is not self-pity. It is not a passive state. This process of daily observation means that you become accountable for your behaviour and take full responsibility for the choices you make. In *The Seven Spiritual Laws of Success,* spiritual leader Deepak Chopra suggests we ask ourselves this question before any action: 'Will the choice I am making bring greater happiness to me and those around me?' This inquiry moves you from reacting to responding. Your self-compassion creates genuine compassion for those you love. You don't try to control or fix them – you offer your presence and love. You stay with the first arrow (remember the Buddhist parable from Week Two) and refrain from creating additional suffering for yourself by adding more arrows through reactivity and obsessive thought patterns.

As you become more mindful in your wakeful state, sleep will emerge easily. When you are walking your dog, you are walking your dog. When you are loading the dishwasher, you are loading the dishwasher. When you are working, you are working. And when you are lying in bed resting, you are lying in bed resting. When you are sleeping, you are sleeping. The body and mind are in the same place at the same time.

Waking Up to a
Higher Consciousness

The morning steals
   upon the night,
Melting the darkness,
   softening light;
The gentle breeze, it
   wakes the flowers,
And whispers to the
   sleeping bowers.

HANNAH MORE

IN THE REALMS of the Eastern spiritual traditions, such as Buddhism, Hinduism and Taoism, lies the profound notion of awakening or enlightenment. These ancient teachings hold a sacred space for the realisation of our true nature, the transcendence of egoic illusions, and the attainment of a higher state of consciousness.

In Buddhism, the term *bodhi* describes the journey towards complete understanding, liberation and freedom from suffering. It is said that Siddhartha Gautama, the historical Buddha, found *bodhi* under the branches of the bodhi tree and was transformed into the awakened one.

In Hinduism, the ultimate reality is known as *Brahman*. This is a process where ignorance is shattered, revealing the direct experience of your divine nature. Under all the layers you wear, you discover the eternal, unchanging essence within yourself, known as *Atman*.

Taoism describes awakening as *wu* – emptiness. The teachings of Taoism advocate simplicity, spontaneity, and the integration of your actions with nature. Taoism recognises your interconnectedness with all things: *I am you; you are me.*

These ancient philosophies teach us to cultivate a sense of peace and harmony within ourselves, with other people and the world. The modern neuroscience of consciousness is beginning to echo these teachings and finally coupling spirituality with science.

The essence of who you are is aliveness, a presence that can easily awaken each day and sleep each night. Call this process *bodhi*, *Brahman* or *wu*, it really doesn't matter. When you begin to awaken, you know it not from its name but from how you perceive your experience of being alive. Fully awakened consciousness becomes the medium by which you experience everything: you see the totality of life and not just a watered-down version.

When asked to describe consciousness to an eight-year-old child, Anil Seth, a globally respected neuroscientist, said, 'It is the redness of red, it is the painfulness of pain, it is the sweetness of honey. It's the fact that everything we do and everything we are — there is something it is like. It feels like something to taste honey, to be happy, to be sad.' He also said, 'It is what makes us more than biological objects roaming around in the subjective dark.'[21] (Which I think was directed more at adults than eight-year-olds!)

As you awaken, you move more slowly and see more sharply. You realise that you don't have to throw multiple arrows at yourself. Life gets easier. You wake up to the essence of your unconditioned self and you naturally sleep serenely. You experience a body and mind that are fully slept, and you learn to nurture and cherish this feeling. You don't find it an effort to make lifestyle choices that support health.

When you find yourself, as we all do, *not* in an awakened state but irritated, anxious, impatient, upset or on edge, this is the time to offer compassion to yourself, not criticism. The spiritual teacher Eckhart Tolle calls these inner disturbances 'the pain body', a set of conditioned emotions that catapult you back into the past. When the pain body arises, which it does, it is an opportunity to observe these transient states, feelings and emotions. Be with them, don't suppress or deny their existence.

As part of my own awakening, an aspect of my own 'pain body' I found exceptionally hard to embrace was jealousy. It's a very ugly emotion to identify with, but I know why it can arise within me. I no longer judge or loathe myself for feeling it. There was a time when feeling jealous was chronic and I had no idea that I felt that way or how it was impacting my relationships. Over the years, my love and awareness have minimised this insecurity greatly. This is liberation. Loving yourself in the moments when you feel most weak and far from perfect is what allows peace, and therefore sleep, to naturally unfold. Give yourself permission to be human and allow any negative feelings to be, and they will no longer disturb you during the day or keep you awake at night.

✦ ✦ ✦

A Collective Awakening

AS MORE PEOPLE awaken on an emotional and spiritual level it is not a coincidence to see that the collective perception of sleep is also changing. The idea that 'sleep is for wimps' or the advice of business tycoons such as Aristotle Onassis, who professed, 'If you sleep three hours less each night for a year, you will have an extra month and a half to succeed,' are thankfully no longer given much heed. Up until

1981, which was when my mother (in her innocence) said, 'You can sleep when you are dead,' there were only 1,292 scientific studies on sleep. By 2022, that number had increased to 24,510.[22]

Classical Greek and Roman civilisations, without any solid scientific data, were very conscious of respecting sleep. Greek dramatist Euripides wrote, 'O dearest charm of sleep, ally against sickness.' In the *Iliad*, Homer calls sleep the 'universal king of gods and men'. The Romans believed that sleep was a gift from the gods and should be cherished and protected.

In the medieval era, particularly in monastic communities, monks and nuns adhered to strict schedules in which rest and sleep were given as much time as prayer and work. There is limited research on the correlation between good sleep and religious belief; one review published in 2018 looked at this connection and, unsurprisingly, found it to be a positive one.[23] The article states, 'Our conceptual model, grounded in the broader religion and health literature, suggests that religious involvement may be associated with healthier sleep outcomes by limiting mental, chemical, and physiological arousal associated with psychological distress, substance use, stress exposure and allostatic load.' Allostatic load refers to the drain that chronic stress has on both the body and the mind. It is also connected to a feeling that one does not have the mental or emotional capacity to meet the demands one has and feels.

People who follow and participate in a religious community tend to have less stress, better social support and a sense of meaning and purpose. All these things lead to a better quality of sleep. You do not have to be religious to cultivate these things; all you need to do is wake up to them. Whether it is through spiritual awakening, scientific enlightenment or a combination of both, sleep is once again getting the respect it deserves. It is time to get intentional, awaken to the healing balm sleep provides, and to restore your vitality and zest for living.

As you read this, I am applying the Sleep Well Formula (Breathe + Imagine + Experience = Faith) on your behalf. Please remember to apply this formula at any stage during the night if you wake up or are disturbed by external challenges (for example, a snoring partner or chronic pain). Accept the situation (if you can't change it) and work through the steps in your mind. The formula is also very effective if you have moments of doubt during your day. If you are in the company of friends or family who are struggling with sleep you can draw on the faith you have found in your ability to sleep well. The formula protects you from absorbing stress and sleep issues that are not yours to carry.

It is my intention to help you sleep. I imagine you now taking conscious deep belly breaths and sleeping peacefully at night, I see you getting to sleep quickly and staying there, I see your relationships improving, I see you laughing, I see you walking into rooms at your work with confidence and grace, I see you navigating situations with ease that in the past caused you high levels of anxiety. I see you and I am already proud. But what matters is whether you can see yourself.

◆ ◆ ◆

A Story of a Yogi: Sat Bir

SAT BIR SINGH KHALSA is an associate professor of medicine in the division of Sleep Medicine at Brigham and Women's Hospital,

Harvard Medical School in Boston. He is also a researcher in the field of mind–body medicine, specialising in research on the efficacy of yoga practices. The combination of Sat Bir's yogic lifestyle and his extensive research on sleep and chronobiology provides the perfect terrain to explore the ingredients required to sleep well.

Sat Bir is aware of the importance of operating from a higher level of consciousness and how each one of us when we awaken contributes to a global awakening. Sat Bir's commitment to both the meditative and the movement practice that yoga teaches leads us to Habit Three this week, 'Move Your Body'. Sat Bir also practises Habit Two, 'Create a "blissful hour" 60-minute bedtime routine', and ensures that he unwinds before sleep. Most of all, what I took from his story is his very straightforward relationship with sleep; he respects it without making a fuss.

I grew up in an immigrant family and there wasn't really any discussion about sleep: you went to bed, you woke up. I currently don't have problems with insomnia; I have a fairly regular bedtime and that manifests into pretty much a regular wake time.

I live in a spiritual yoga community, and I lead some of the morning practices, which begin at 4 a.m. So, on those days, I might wake up a little bit earlier, but I'm already regularly going to bed fairly early.

I don't routinely take a nap. I would only take a nap if I'd had a temporary sleep disturbance or had to stay up late, or had to get up particularly early. My energy is steady and I'm not fighting drowsiness during the day or carrying any sleep debt on a regular basis. I like to get the full amount of sleep because I am cognisant of the importance of it for virtually every function in the body. I'm therefore very respectful of my need for sleep.

My expertise in sleep has come largely through studying sleep and chronobiology as an academic and a researcher starting in 1985. Although my hope and ultimate goal was to conduct research in yoga and meditative states of consciousness, there were no opportunities for that at that time, so I had to find some field of research that perhaps had some degree of relevance to that goal. Of course, sleep is a state of consciousness, and so at least I would be studying the regulation of states of consciousness. I began research in the field of chronobiology (the study of biological rhythms), first with an animal model, and then, when I moved to Harvard, working on human sleep and chronobiological characteristics.

When the National Center for Complementary and Integrative Health (which funds research on mind–body practices such as yoga) started funding full grants that would support a salary, and with my yoga expertise and my training in sleep and chronobiology, I was in a position to acquire funding and conduct studies of yoga for chronic insomnia.

Every organism on the planet has evolved in a 24-hour day–night cycle and, as a consequence, all organisms are wired at the genetic level for daily changes in activity. In higher organisms this manifests as a sleep–wake cycle. Sleep is a natural process. It's not something that you can wilfully make happen; it's something that happens to you when you create the right circumstances and everything is aligned appropriately.

There's a significant influence of behavioural conditioning involved in our sleep characteristics and habits. If you go to bed at 2 a.m. one night and then 9 p.m. the next night and vary your sleep schedule substantially, that may prevent stable conditioning and appropriate synchronisation of your biological clock to the day–night cycle from happening, which could contribute to a sleep problem. Consuming alcohol as a sleep aid will help you to fall asleep, but it will disturb the quality and depth of your sleep and might precipitate early morning awakenings. With regular alcohol use, there is also the risk of a substance abuse problem.

There are a lot of sleep hygiene practices that are well known in sleep medicine, most of which are common-sense recommendations – for example, have a comfortable bed and bedroom, keep it dark, keep the temperature appropriate, and keep the noise down. However, surprisingly, some people just don't implement them adequately.

With respect to sleep need and sleep duration, different individuals may have different needs based on their inherited genetic makeup. Most adults need seven-and-a-half to eight hours of sleep. There are relatively few people who require much less or much more sleep.

One characteristic that can affect sleep is personality type. People who tend to have more anxious personalities are more prone to sleep disturbance. It doesn't mean if you are anxious you are necessarily going to have sleep disturbance, but it may mean you are more prone to it. This also applies to any other mental or physical dysfunction or disorder because virtually every disease has some negative impact on sleep. However, even people who have challenges with sleep or risk factors for sleep disturbance can do things to enhance their sleep quality through behavioural interventions such as the sleep hygiene recommendations described above.

As a sleep researcher and someone who's had clinical experience with sleep disorders, I know the importance of incorporating a wind-down time as another important sleep hygiene recommendation. You don't just do your taxes and your accounting until 9 p.m. and then hop into bed at 9.01 p.m. and expect to fall asleep. It's best to engage in an hour or two of some kind of non-stressful activity that allows you to glide into the circumstances that are conducive to sleep, which includes a lower level of mental and physical arousal. Sleep needs to have some degree of relaxation and calmness and a lower level of stress and anxiety. If you are experiencing some degree of stress and anxiety due to an upcoming life event such as an exam or a court case, your stress system is more activated and you need to take steps to calm your system in order to get a deeper quality of sleep for the full night.

Sleep will be disturbed with acute levels of arousal but also with what we call chronic sustained stress. Chronic stress is known to be negatively affecting well over a third of the US population. Chronic stress will likely translate into lighter or disturbed sleep and in some cases overt and full-blown clinical insomnia.

We have fairly strong scientific evidence that most people who have chronic insomnia show elevated levels of psychophysiological arousal of the stress systems. This means a higher sympathetic drive, with higher sympathetic nerve activation and higher levels of adrenaline associated with higher heart rate and lower heart rate variability. Levels of the stress hormone cortisol are also chronically higher. This has led to the characterisation of the hyperarousal hypothesis of insomnia, that it's the increased psychophysiological arousal that keeps people from getting a good night's sleep. From this perspective, insomnia is not a sleep disorder; it's a disorder of arousal. Therefore, if you reduce this arousal, you are likely to improve sleep quality.

A classic example of this is caffeine, which is an arousing agent. It works on the neurotransmitter adenosine, so if you drink a lot of caffeine it's going to take you longer to fall asleep, your sleep will be lighter, and you might wake up earlier. You can actually mimic insomnia by ingesting high levels of caffeine throughout the day.

One of the biggest and most immediate benefits of yoga is the reduction in psychophysiological arousal by reducing activation of the stress systems. If you begin to regularly practise yoga, you will reduce the sympathetic drive and enhance parasympathetic activity, lower stress hormone levels, and improve the ability to regulate emotional reactivity more effectively. As a consequence, you will likely improve sleep quality.

People who have chronic insomnia are often caught in a vicious cycle. They ruminate about their insomnia, and experience dysfunctional and counterproductive thoughts around sleep. This occurs especially during mid-sleep awakenings in which these thought patterns keep them tossing and turning and thinking about how bad their sleep is. Of course, these dysfunctional thoughts are actually exacerbating the problem. A solution to this is to improve regulation of thought processes.

The meditative practices in yoga train you to improve self-regulation over your thought processes. You become more of a master of your mind and thoughts. This allows you to become less reactive to arousing thoughts. Ultimately, meditative practices lead to the realisation that you are not your thoughts, a state referred to as metacognition. In a formal behavioural intervention that is effective for insomnia called cognitive behavioural therapy, you learn to identify dysfunctional thoughts and replace them with neutral thoughts, and thereby also come to the experience of metacognition.

Personally, if I wake too early or in the middle of the night, reading a book is typically enough for me to relax and get out of any negative rumination and fall back asleep. However, there are some very specific yoga practices that I can do that can help me get back to sleep. One of those is called bridge pose and I find that that it's often effective to help me get back to sleep. Bridge pose has been recommended in a number of different yoga traditions as being good for sleep, so there's some commonality historically for that belief.

Insomnia treatment largely consists of removing the things that are preventing sleep, and modern behavioural treatments are actually very effective. Once you clear up the dysfunctional behaviours or the secondary causes of insomnia, the vast majority of people are going to revert back to normal sleep.

Build Your Sleep Well Habits

PLEASE CONTINUE WITH the habits you've formed in the previous weeks. Remember that we are not looking for perfection. Some days will be better than others. On the days that you practise your habits, acknowledge your progress. On the days you don't, be compassionate to yourself and resolve to continue with them the next day. No pressure.

HABIT THREE

Move Your Body

Movement is a medicine for creating change in a person's physical, emotional, and mental states.

CAROL WELCH

ONE OF THE places I love to go on retreat to write and reflect is Glenstal Abbey, a Benedictine monastery that welcomes guests no matter what religious beliefs you have or don't have. It is a very spiritual place and one where my sleep is always very deep. On a recent visit, I asked Father Christopher, the guest master, if he was a good sleeper. He seemed surprised by my question. 'Of course,' he replied.

'What's your secret?' I asked.

'A good day's work. I always sleep well because I work hard.'

When I asked him if he meant sitting in his office on a computer, again he seemed surprised. 'No, physical,' he said. 'I am busy moving all day.'

As the housekeeper of the guest house, Father Christopher is often on his feet, taking care of guests and making sure everything is running smoothly. He also spends several hours a day singing at Mass and Vespers. Father Christopher reported that he wasn't aware of any sleep issues in the monastery, which has a population of almost forty monks; he did say that only one or two of the very elderly monks mentioned their sleep being disturbed on occasion.

Physical work coupled with a spiritual life leads to a good night's sleep. Like the birth of electricity, the introduction of a sedentary lifestyle has played havoc with our sleep. You were born to move, walk for hours, stretch, carry weight, all through the necessity of hunting and foraging for your food. Once your belly was full and the sun was high in the sky, you rested. All of these behaviours afforded you the ease of a good night's sleep as soon as the light of the day began to fade and the stars started to shine.

You were designed to be in touch with and to move with nature.

In the modern era, many people drive or commute to work or walk to their home office and sit for most of their day. Almost all jobs, even active ones, require people to spend some time on a computer every day. To add to this, much of our leisure time is also sedentary, whether we're watching TV, scrolling the internet or playing video games.

Leading a sedentary lifestyle is associated with various negative health outcomes, including obesity, type 2 diabetes, cardiovascular diseases, and certain types of cancer, and it can intensify depression and anxiety. Sedentary behaviour has also been associated with musculoskeletal issues, such as back pain and reduced muscle strength and flexibility.

The latest research shows that globally more than 80 per cent of adolescents and 27 per cent of adults do not meet the World Health Organization (WHO) recommended levels of physical activity.[24] These recommendations are, to my mind, very achievable for most people in reasonable health: adults aged 18–64 years should do at least 150–300 minutes of moderate-intensity aerobic physical activity per week (this is only an average of 20–40 minutes per day) or at least 75–150 minutes of vigorous-intensity aerobic physical activity; or an equivalent combination of moderate- and vigorous-intensity activity throughout the week.

What level of movement are you getting per day? The above guidelines are specifically for focused exercises such as going for a run, going to the gym, a yoga class or playing a sport. However, it is worth noting how much time you spend moving, hoovering, changing beds and climbing stairs, all examples of informal exercise. Don't underestimate how much you are already moving!

The benefits of moving your body and getting exercise every day include overall improved quality, sleep latency (time to get to sleep), sleep duration, and the ability to stay asleep. Exercise has also been shown to help alleviate sleep apnoea due to a reduction in weight. It also affects the structure of your sleep stages, with an increase in slow-wave deep sleep and an enhancement in REM sleep quality. It is also well documented that exercise alleviates symptoms of anxiety and depression, which will in turn help you to feel calmer and have a lower level of arousal before sleep.

WHAT TIME IS BEST TO EXERCISE FOR SLEEP?
To maximise your sleep quality, it is recommended that you exercise as soon as you can after rising. Timing exercise with your sunlight exposure is ideal.

If this is not enough to tempt you up and out first thing, there are also studies that show exercising on an empty stomach before breakfast burns up to 20 per cent more body fat than exercising after breakfast.[25] Early morning exercise can also boost self-esteem, as you will naturally feel good about yourself as you progress during the day knowing that you have already started it on a healthy footing.

If your schedule simply does not allow for early morning exercise, there are also some benefits to afternoon and evening exercise, such as your reaction time being faster, which can be good for team sports and high-intensity workouts.[26] The late afternoon is also when your heart rate and blood pressure are lowest, which decreases your chance of injury while improving performance.

It was once recommended that you avoid exercising in the evening at all costs; however, Harvard University recently conducted a meta-analysis that indicates exercising in the evening no later than one hour before bed (and as long as it is not too high intensity) can help you to fall and stay asleep.[27] If you exercise later in the day, a hot shower will help you to reduce your core body temperature. As with all of the habits in this programme, you will find what works best for you.

What this Looks Like for Me

I 'formally' exercise six out of seven days with a combination of yoga, running and swimming. I generally move first thing in the morning and in the summer I exercise outside in the sunlight and in winter I combine exercise with light therapy.

I move as much as I can during the day. While working at home I intersperse periods of sitting/standing at the computer with household chores. I get up and water the plants or unload the dishwasher. Also, I like to go out for a walk (weather permitting) at lunchtime and/or in the evening. It is not perfect, and some days, especially while writing a book, I am sedentary for way too long. Please remember you are aiming for a strategy that is realistic for your life and health circumstances.

The movement that has really uplifted my heart and soul and helped me to feel strong physically and emotionally is my regular yoga practice. I started dabbling with yoga in my early twenties but have become a 'serious' practitioner in the last ten years. Along with hypnotherapy and meditation, yoga has transformed my life and sleep. I practise mainly vinyasa flow and ashtanga but will lean towards yin and restorative practices when I feel the need to reduce my stress levels. In the winter, a hot yoga class can be great for relaxing muscles. I do a 60-minute class a minimum of three times a week and find myself in a down dog at some stage most days. I really notice the difference when I fall out of this routine due to travel or work commitments: my body is stiff, and my emotions are less regulated. I am known to look for a yoga studio no matter where I am. I prefer to practise in person but will use an app or video to supplement my classes. One of my teachers says, 'You practise to become stronger so that you can be stronger for others.' I feel this strength emotionally but also physically when I travel with my husband – he is grateful that he no longer needs to carry my case up or down stairs.

Thanks to pioneers such as Dr Sat Bir Singh Khalsa and other researchers in the field of yoga, we now have the evidence that supports what yoga practitioners have known on a subjective and anecdotal level for thousands of years.

If you practise yoga regularly, you will sleep better.

The origins of yoga can be traced back over 5,000 years to ancient India. The word 'yoga' is derived from the Sanskrit word 'yuj,' which means to unite or join. Yoga is not just a form of exercise; it offers you a way to live in harmony with yourself, others and the world. Consider it a technology for inner well-being that is accessible to everyone regardless of their age, culture or background.

A traditional yoga class has three components that elevate physical, spiritual and mental well-being. These are meditation (metacognition), pranayama (breath control) and asanas (yoga postures and flow). A skilled teacher will guide your nervous system on a journey that mirrors the 24-hour wake–sleep circadian cycle. You start off in a low state of arousal with meditation, and you then do pranayama breath work, which slightly elevates your arousal, before moving into the moving asanas (poses) which activate your sympathetic nervous system and increase your levels of cortisol, then things slow down again before ending up in shavasana (the corpse pose), which requires total surrender.

Your afternoon resting ritual audio included in the Sleep Well audios is a beautiful example of this. Yoga teaches you how to regulate your nervous system to suit what level of arousal is appropriate for the time of day and activity you are engaged in.

Yoga increases your vagal tone (the activity level of your vagus nerve) and lowers your heart rate, which will minimise the time it takes sleep to come. In one study on older people, a yoga intervention of six months helped the participants to get to sleep faster, improved the quality of their sleep and saw an overall reduction in the use of sleeping pills. This cohort also reported feeling more refreshed when they woke compared to the group who did not practise yoga.[28]

On the other side of the scale, a Swedish study on young adult students showed that those who practised yoga for six weeks at a frequent and intense level showed an improvement in the quality of their sleep.[29]

Yoga is also very effective for emotional regulation which, as you know, helps you to sleep. In many of the asanas (poses), you release a build-up of tension and emotion that is stored in the body. The hip-opening exercises are particularly effective at releasing emotional pain. The discipline of regular practice develops concentration, focus, resilience and self-awareness.

Bessel van der Kolk, psychiatrist and best-selling author of the iconic book *The Body Keeps the Score*, recommends yoga as an intervention that is far more effective than any medication. It is the feeling of connection and safety that we cultivate through yoga that helps us to occupy our bodies without anxiety, he says: 'Self-regulation depends on having a friendly relationship with your body. Without it, you have to rely on external regulation – from medication, drugs like alcohol, constant reassurance, or compulsive compliance with the wishes of others.'

There are six main types of yoga. It can be confusing when you first start (and even when you are a seasoned practitioner) to know which one is best suited to your needs. They are:

Hatha Yoga
Hatha yoga is a general term that encompasses various physical postures (asanas) and breathing techniques (pranayama). It is practised at a slower pace, focusing on alignment and balance. It helps to improve flexibility and strength.

Vinyasa Yoga
Also known as flow yoga, it is characterised by fluid and continuous movements that synchronise breath with movement. It involves transitioning from one pose to another in a flowing sequence. Vinyasa yoga improves cardiovascular health, builds strength, and enhances body awareness and coordination.

Ashtanga Yoga

Ashtanga yoga is a dynamic and physically demanding practice that follows a specific sequence of poses. It incorporates synchronised breathing and movement, and each pose is held for a specific number of breaths. Ashtanga yoga builds strength, stamina and flexibility, while also promoting mental focus and discipline.

Kundalini Yoga

Kundalini yoga combines dynamic movements, breathing techniques, chanting and meditation to awaken dormant spiritual energy within the body known as kundalini. It aims to balance the mind, body, and spirit and promote self-awareness, intuition and inner transformation.

Yin Yoga

Yin yoga involves holding passive poses for an extended period, typically three to five minutes. It targets the deep connective tissues, ligaments and joints, improving flexibility and increasing circulation. It has a calming and meditative effect, promoting relaxation and mindfulness. It is also useful for building resilience and acceptance of life's challenges and for releasing emotion from the body.

Restorative Yoga

Restorative yoga focuses on deep relaxation and stress relief. It involves the use of props to support the body in gentle, comfortable poses, allowing for complete relaxation and restoration. Restorative yoga promotes a sense of calm, reduces anxiety, and helps in healing and rejuvenation. Really good to practise if you are going through a hard time such as grief or divorce.

These are the most common styles offered, but you will find hot yoga and aerial yoga too. I have also heard of laughter yoga, which I would love to try! My sister, who lives in Berlin, recently saw a naked yoga class being advertised – I am not so sure about that one! Each style offers unique benefits, but they all share the goal of uniting your body and mind. It's important to choose a style that suits your needs, preferences and physical capabilities. If you already have a regular yoga practice, I am speaking to the converted; you will know how incredibly beneficial it is for your overall well-being. If not, would you consider beginning one? Yoga is not for everyone and many people find it a challenge to stay present during the class. If so, I recommend you commit to at least six months before deciding it is not for you.

A POSE TO PRACTISE TONIGHT

Practise before bed, and again if you wake up at night or in the early morning and need an extra helping hand to get back to sleep. As the name suggests, the pose looks like the shape of a bridge. The purpose of the pose is to open your chest, heart and shoulders. It creates a lovely stretch at the back of the neck, the thighs and the hip flexors. It is known, as Sat Bir said, to help induce sleep and also provides relief from stress, fatigue, anxiety and mild headaches. Avoid this pose if you have a neck or shoulder injury.

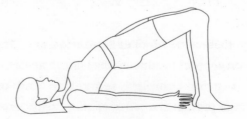

1 **Lie on your back**, bending knees and centring yourself on the mat. Point knees to the sky with feet flat on the ground.

2 **Adjust arms and feet**, palms facing down, extending arms sideways. Keep feet hip-width apart and fingertips grazing heels.

3 **Lift hips** by pressing down through feet and hands without squeezing glutes.

4 **Tuck chin slightly** to lengthen the back of your neck.

5 **Interlace hands behind your back**, inch shoulder blades beneath you, and lift torso while pressing hands down.

6 **Relax glutes**, engage inner thighs, and breathe steadily.

7 **Lift hips higher briefly**, feeling the stretch in the lower back and hip flexors.

8 **Breathe deeply** in this position for one minute.

9 **Slowly release** by unlacing fingers and lowering hips and your back, vertebra by vertebra, until the tailbone touches the floor. Take deep breaths to conclude the pose.

10 **Repeat as necessary** – three times is good before bed or if you wake up too early.

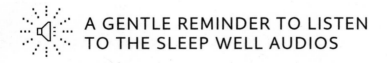# A GENTLE REMINDER TO LISTEN TO THE SLEEP WELL AUDIOS

You can access these audios for FREE with the passcode ISLEEPWELL on www.thepositivehabit.com.

Please remember to listen to the instructions for listening to guarantee maximum benefits.

MORNING MEDITATION

Please listen each morning to 'Start Your Day in Stillness – Intention-Setting Morning Meditation' to slow down your thoughts, before the day commences.

AFTERNOON OR EVENING REST RITUAL

Please listen to 'Seven-Minute Rest Ritual' each afternoon and/or evening.

NIGHT-TIME HYPNOTHERAPY – WEEK THREE: HABIT THREE

This is the most important track to listen to. Each week there are new subconscious suggestions to help to reinforce the corresponding weekly habit and the following key insights.

TO GET BACK TO SLEEP IF YOU WAKE UP

You can listen to your night-time audio again, if necessary, but with time you will not need to do this. The Sleep Well Formula (Breathe + Imagine + Experience = Faith) which you are learning on a subconscious level every time you listen to your weekly audios will become automatic. Please also listen to the '4, 7, 8 Breathing' audio and train yourself to do this in the middle of the night should you awaken.

THE GOLDEN KEY INSIGHTS FROM WEEK THREE: YOUR WAKING SELF

✦ The practice of formal sitting meditation (your morning audio and rest ritual) and informal mindfulness (moment-to-moment awareness) are doorways to observe, understand and love your unconditioned self.

✦ My three-step mindfulness tool ARC (Accept, Release and Compassion) is a highly practical and powerful mindfulness tool to let go of unnecessary fear and emotional pain as it arises.

- When you are awake and idle your mind will inevitably wander. In this state, the default mode network (DMN) is activated. Mind wandering has positive outcomes such as creative insights and greater clarity on decision-making. However, living permanently in this state is a block to presence and connecting to yourself, others and the world around you. The formal and informal practices mentioned above will help you to become more present.

- The essence of who you are is aliveness, a presence that can easily awaken each day and sleep each night. Call this process *bodhi*, *Brahman* or *wu*, it really doesn't matter. When you begin to awaken, you know it not from its name but from how you perceive your experience of being alive.

- Can you begin to see and imagine yourself sleeping peacefully at night, getting to sleep quickly and staying there, your relationships improving, laughing, walking into rooms at your work with confidence and grace, navigating situations with ease that in the past caused you high levels of anxiety? Remember your Sleep Well Formula: Breathe + Imagine + Experience = Faith.

- Habit Three is 'Move Your Body'.

To maximise the benefits of this programme, I encourage you not to begin reading Week Four until you have listened to the 'Week Three: Habit Three' night-time audio for a minimum of seven nights in total.

Remember, your sleep story is not finished and is always a work in progress. Keep going! Please remember to acknowledge all progress with your habits and mindset, no matter how big or small.

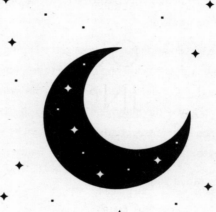

YOUR
SLEEPING SELF

Your subconscious never sleeps. It is always on the job. It controls all your vital functions. Forgive yourself and everyone else before you go to sleep, and healing will take place much more rapidly

JOSEPH MURPHY, *THE POWER OF YOUR SUBCONSCIOUS MIND*

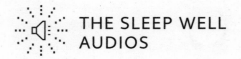

THE SLEEP WELL AUDIOS

All audios are available to download on www.thepositivehabit.com with the password ISLEEPWELL.

✦ Tonight, please start listening to 'Week Four: Habit Four' of your Sleep Well audios. Please listen to this audio for a minimum of seven nights. Please do not skip ahead to Week Five until you have listened for a full seven days.

✦ Please also continue to listen to your morning meditation and your rest ritual tracks each day.

✦ ✦ ✦

Measure Your Sleep

BEFORE YOU BEGIN Week Four of the Sleep Well Programme, please take a moment to rate your sleep. On a scale of 0 to 10, how well have you slept in the last week? (0 is 'terribly' and 10 is 'very well'.) Please use the image on the opposite page to mark where you feel you are on this scale.

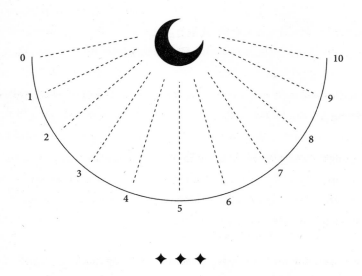

✦ ✦ ✦

Welcome to Week Four

HOW ARE YOU getting on? I truly hope you're doing well. It is essential to take each night as it comes and remember you are not seeking perfect sleep every night because, well, it doesn't exist and therefore it is unattainable. What is very possible, and what we are working towards, is that you reach your own sleeping potential. This differs for all of us depending on the stage of our life and external triggers. For example, if you currently have a young baby, you are most certainly not getting the best sleep of your life. But with the Sleep Well Programme, you will be ensuring that it is as effective as it can be considering your circumstances.

This week is fascinating as we take a deeper dive into the subconscious mind – this time, when you are asleep. I will expand on the most up-to-date science on neuroplasticity and how to maximise your brain's capacity to change itself. We will explore the five stages of sleep and why each one plays a critical role in the overall effectiveness of your sleep. I will further help you with the all-important question of how to get back to sleep if/when you wake in the middle of the night or early morning; you are already practising your Sleep Well Formula to help you with this each night in your audios. We will explore the world of dreams and the role they play in regulating your emotions. We will also look at lucid dreaming and nightmares and, of course, I have a brand-new habit for you to build. Enjoy and keep going.

Sleep and the Subconscious in Our First Seven Years

WHEN I WAS a young child, about five or six, I had a doll called Strawberry Shortcake. I loved this doll so much and believed she came to life while I slept. I can still recall the sweet (albeit fake) smell of strawberries from her skin that never seemed to fade. For a time, I wrote to her every night and would leave her my precious ration of Jaffa cakes at the end of my bed for her to eat while I slept. I would wait as long as I could to see her wake up, but I always fell asleep before she appeared. Every morning when I woke, the Jaffa cakes were miraculously eaten and there was a reply from Strawberry Shortcake, thanking me for my generosity. The friendship we had formed made me feel so special. I had a doll that came alive – just for me.

For the first seven years of life, theta is the predominant brainwave state that we live in (brainwaves are patterns of electrical activity generated by the brain). Theta is also present in adults in the onset of sleep, deep relaxation, creativity, enhanced learning, deep meditation and, in particular, hypnosis. The magical moments just before you slip into sleep are pure gold when it comes to neuroplastic shifts in your subconscious mind as your brain enters theta and your subconscious mind is most malleable.[30]

Theta brainwaves allow us to access the power of the subconscious mind and are also often associated with heightened intuition, increased visualisation and a sense of spiritual connection. In this state, your imagination is wide open, and the world is full of constant wonder. When your mind wanders as you drift to sleep into disconnected and random images and thoughts, this is the door of your sleeping subconscious self-opening. It is important to allow the mind to wander in this state, let it roam. The difference between the conscious mind and the subconscious in this transitory state before sleep is that the conscious mind will be thinking about what you have to do the next day and the subconscious is fuelled solely by the imagination: the thoughts and images often don't have much logic to them, just like a dream.

As a child, you may have wanted to be an astronaut or the president, and you didn't doubt yourself or the endless possibilities of what you could be. You probably, like me, believed dolls came alive at night. (You wouldn't have suspected it was your big sister who loved Jaffa cakes!) Children live in an almost permanent state of hypnosis. They are downloading information rather than actively trying to learn it, hence the idea that their brains are like sponges. At this age, neuroplastic change is experience-led and fast.[31] The human brain doubles in size in the first year of life. By age three, it is forming one million neural connections each minute.

Dr Bruce Lipton, developmental biologist and author of *The Biology of Belief*, says that 'ninety-five per cent of our current choices and circumstances are coming from the programs of life that we receive in the first seven years of our childhood'. You did not choose these programs; they were chosen for you by the adults in your life, society at large, and your cultural conditioning. As you learned last week, it is possible that you downloaded unhelpful beliefs about your capacity to sleep well. Now that you are questioning them you will refrain from passing them on to the next generation. Hallelujah!

Often, there is a mix of positive learnings coupled with less-than-perfect examples that could be creating confusion in your life today. For example, if you had a parent who was both quick-tempered and also very physically affectionate, you may find it hard to know how to relate to figures of authority in your life today. As we explored in Week Two, the story you tell yourself matters. Humans are a mix of both dark and light. You need to select the programs you wish to prune and those you wish to nourish.

In order for this to happen, you need to access the brain state in which those early programs were first formed – theta. Adult neuroplasticity needs to be self-directed, and it requires repetition to be able to change from one emotional state to another. To let go of a negative belief or to learn a new task, you need to repeat something until it becomes automatic. For example, driving a car, riding a bike or learning an instrument all take significant conscious awareness when you first learn them. After a time, though, these skills require less effort and are ingrained into your muscle memory and the neural pathways of your brain.

The subconscious, like a child,

✦ Takes everything you say literally

✦ Does not distinguish negative from positive

✦ Does not distinguish reality from imagination

✦ Has no sense of irony

✦ Obeys authority

✦ Requires consistent guidance and reassurance

✦ Is slow to change

✦ Thrives on routine

✦ Reads emotions as facts

✦ Wants to please you

When communicating with your subconscious, keep your language simple and positive. It will serve you well once you feed it with nurturing thoughts. For example, when you say in your own mind or out loud, 'I can't cope with another bad night's sleep,' the subconscious hears bad + night + sleep. It is like a vegetarian going into a restaurant, ordering a steak and getting annoyed with the waiter when they bring meat. The connection between you and sleep is now a negative one. Your subconscious received this thought as a command and understands that you are requesting a bad night's sleep. Recall our work in Week Two again, on becoming a non-complaining good sleeper.

Neuroplasticity and Sleep

There is one protocol that has been shown by the greatest number of scientific studies to produce not just states of deep relaxation, not just states of heightened focus but also to accelerate plasticity and learning in the brain and that is hypnosis.

ANDREW HUBERMAN, NEUROSCIENTIST
AND PROFESSOR AT STANFORD UNIVERSITY

YOUR HYPNOTHERAPY AUDIO will glide you gently into the theta brainwave state. The audios also encompass your Sleep Well Formula: Breathe + Imagine + Experience = Faith. Consider hypnotherapy as yoga for the mind; it requires consistent practice to obtain maximum strength and flexibility.

Neuroplastic changes occur when you sleep rather than at the time of learning.

Sleep resets brain connections, it processes the day's information and consolidates new information that it deems to be vital for your survival. Giulio Tononi, a neuroscientist and psychiatrist who holds the David P. White Chair in Sleep Medicine at the University of Wisconsin-Madison, says, 'Learning and memory require synaptic activity, which is very energetically expensive and prone to saturation. Sleep allows the brain to renormalise this synaptic activity after it increases in the waking day.'[32]

In addition to helping you reconnect with your innate ability to sleep, the hypnosis audios are carving your three core sleep strengths into your brain: presence, patience and peace. As you listen repetitively, you are downloading new programs into your subconscious as you drift to sleep. These are then marinating in your neural networks as you drift in and out of the five stages of sleep.

✦ ✦ ✦

The Five Stages of Sleep

SLEEP IS NOT a static state. Sleep scientists have recently classified the main sleep stages you need to move through to optimise the effectiveness of your sleep over an 8-hour sleep opportunity. Each stage has its unique set of functions and benefits, which are listed below.

Sleep latency is the amount of time it takes to get to sleep from the moment you turn off the light and close your eyes. This time varies from person to person and depends on your age, sleep hygiene, sleep challenges (either chronic or acute) and environmental conditions. Matthew Walker, the renowned sleep researcher mentioned earlier, says a healthy individual should ideally fall asleep within 15 to 20 minutes of closing their eyes. Your sleep audios will assist you in this period. However, if you are not asleep by the end of the audio, don't despair. Continue to focus on the idea that you are resting rather than 'trying' to sleep.

Sleep architecture is the term used to describe the sleep journey from beginning to end. Each sleep cycle lasts roughly 90–120 minutes and the number you have can vary from four to six each night. Everyone will have a unique pattern, yet none of us can skip a stage.

For the purpose of this book, I am adding an initial sleep stage. A bold move, I know, but adding an initial pre-sleep stage ensures the other four are reached more easily.

STAGE ONE: PRE-SLEEP (30–60 MINS)

Not officially a stage of sleep, as you are still awake! However, allocating time to begin the relaxation process is imperative for the overall quality of your night's sleep. A bedtime routine that cues safety will encourage a smooth transition into sleep. For example, if you want to be asleep by 11.00 pm, the process of going to bed needs to start by 10 p.m. You will be practising this already from Week Two: Habit Two (the 'blissful hour' bedtime routine) and, I am sure, feeling the benefits. A bedtime routine aimed at helping your brain move from alpha brainwave (which is associated with an awake, yet relaxed, state) towards theta brainwave will ensure you give yourself every opportunity to get to sleep and stay asleep.

Benefits: Slows down the mind, cleanses and clears stress, activates the parasympathetic nervous system and encourages the transition to sleep.

STAGE TWO: TRANSITIONING TO SLEEP – 5 PER CENT–10 PER CENT OF TIME SPENT IN AN 8-HOUR SLEEP OPPORTUNITY

The lights are off and the initial onset of sleep is commencing: your brain is now in the malleable theta brainwave. You are drifting between the two states of wakefulness and light sleep. Your eye movements are slow.

Benefits: Relaxation and surrendering from your waking world.

STAGE THREE: LIGHT SLEEP – 45 PER CENT–55 PER CENT OF TIME SPENT IN AN 8-HOUR SLEEP OPPORTUNITY

Deeper than stage two. Brain wave patterns include short bursts of rapid brain activity known as sleep spindles. Eye movements cease, and your body temperature decreases.

Benefits: Consolidation of memory and preparation for deep sleep stages.

STAGE FOUR: DEEP SLEEP – NON-RAPID EYE MOVEMENT (NREM) – 15 PER CENT–25 PER CENT OF TIME SPENT IN AN 8-HOUR SLEEP OPPORTUNITY

The deepest stage, characterised by the appearance of slow, high-amplitude delta waves. The benefits of this stage of sleep are bountiful; here are the main ones.

+ **Cognitive function:** the transfer of information from short-term memory to long-term memory, resulting in the retention and recall of learned material.

+ **Emotional regulation:** reduces the emotional intensity associated with negative experiences, making them easier to cope with and regulate during wakefulness.

+ **Metabolic regulation:** balancing of hormones related to appetite, hunger and energy regulation.

+ **Cardiovascular health:** helps regulate blood pressure, reduces inflammation, and promotes a healthy balance of blood sugar levels.

+ **Immune system support:** promotes the production of immune cells and antibodies to help fight off infections and diseases.

- ✦ **Restores mental energy:** allows you to concentrate and focus.

- ✦ **Detoxification and waste clearance:** also known as the dishwasher of the brain, deep sleep clears waste products from the brain, including harmful substances like beta-amyloid, which is associated with the development of Alzheimer's disease.

STAGE FIVE: REM SLEEP – 20 PER CENT–25 PER CENT OF TIME SPENT IN AN 8-HOUR SLEEP OPPORTUNITY

Eye movement becomes rapid, and you enter the dreaming state. In this state, your brain has increased activity that is similar to wakefulness, and your muscles are temporarily paralysed to ensure that you do not act out your dreams. REM cycles get longer as the night goes on and are more dominant in the second half of the night, increasing in duration each time. Often the longest one is active just before you wake up.

Benefits: Memory consolidation, emotional processing and regulation, creativity, learning, and overall cognitive functioning.

The most helpful thing to do if you wake up in the middle of a cycle is to remind yourself that you are simply in a lighter phase of sleep. Lighter phases increase in the second four hours of the night. We all experience them. Accepting that lighter sleep is normal and that there is no need to interfere with the natural architecture of your sleep will help you immensely.

If you get up in the middle of a cycle, you are interrupting the pattern, and it cannot be compensated for at another time. For example, deciding to go to the gym at 5 a.m. one morning, when you usually wake at 6.30 a.m., means you will miss your final REM cycle. Your dreams not only play a crucial role in your emotional regulation but also contain a lot of wisdom to help you reach your potential in your waking world.

How to Get Back to Sleep if You Wake Up

If you wake up in the middle of the night or early in the morning, please apply the Sleep Well Formula silently to yourself in your mind. The sooner you intervene before the conscious mind takes full control, the faster you will return to a deeper sleep. In other words, you make a conscious decision not to engage your conscious mind, for example by getting frustrated at being awake. **It is essential that you do not check the time** as this will ignite a higher level of arousal, the very thing you do not want. The time can take care of itself. Even if you have to be up in 20 minutes, it is 20 minutes' more rest to enjoy rather than 20 minutes to get stressed. Resist this temptation – it is so worth it.

> **Being patient with yourself in these moments will ease any frustration.**

As soon as you notice that you are in a lighter phase of sleep, please follow these steps.

1   Accept that it is normal.

2   Begin the formula and begin to **breathe** deeply into your belly.

3   **Imagine** a beautiful place you find relaxing; it could be from the Sleep Well night-time hypnotherapy audio, or a place you love and have been to many times.

4   **Experience** the joy of resting and the comfort of your bed, and recall how many times you have effortlessly got back to sleep in the past.

5   Have **faith** that sleep will return when the time is right. Be patient and focus on resting, not trying to get back to sleep.

If you still find yourself awake and in an anxious state after 15 or 20 minutes, you can choose to put your audio back on. This option is only for extreme cases if you feel you need the guidance – perhaps you are going through a very tough time or your mind is spinning. Above all, trust yourself that you can allow sleep to return. The beauty is that once you have done it yourself a few times, it becomes second nature and a reliable resource for you to draw on. If I wake up in the early hours, I choose to imagine something from my day in detail: the trees outside my window, the view to the sea on my walk. It's very accessible and soothing and before I know it sleep has gracefully returned and I am back in the magical land of my dreams.

✦ ✦ ✦

The Enigma of Dreams

Hold fast to dreams
For if dreams die
Life is a broken-winged bird
That cannot fly.

LANGSTON HUGHES (1901–1967)

THE FASCINATION WITH the enigma of dreams began back in the world's oldest civilisations. The ancient Egyptians and Greeks both believed that dreams conveyed important messages from the gods. The god Horus in ancient Egypt was believed to directly communicate with people through their dreams with words of wisdom that helped to protect the sleeper in their waking world. The Greek philosophers Aristotle and Plato both preached the principle that dreams offered insights into a person's psyche and emotions, and could predict future events.

In the late nineteenth century, Sigmund Freud, the father of the subconscious mind, introduced his psychoanalytic theory of dreams. Freud used dream interpretation as the prime method to access the hidden desires and repressed emotions of his patients. These desires, he believed, were often sexual in nature. Freud's Oedipus and Electra complexes suggests that children hold latent sexual desires for their parents of the opposite gender, and hence see the parent of the same sex as a rival. This view was, and still remains, controversial.

Carl Jung, a Swiss psychiatrist who was heavily influenced by the work of Freud, saw things differently. Jung deemed Freud's theory of sexual repression too reductionist; he believed that our dreams offer us a greater understanding of ourselves and also a wider view into the collective unconscious. The collective unconscious, according to Jung, is a deeper level of the mind that all human beings share, regardless of their cultural conditioning. It is an innate instinct that is inherited from one generation by the next in the form of archetypes rather than through personal experience. Jung believed that an understanding of how these archetypes impact the individual would lead to a greater sense of psychological harmony and wholeness.

Dream interpretation was deemed important by ancient Western cultures right through to the Middle Ages and beyond through Christianity, with priests and religious figures interpreting the possible hidden messages in the dreams of their followers. However, with the Age of Enlightenment and the birth of modern science, less and less significance (apart from the work of psychoanalysts) has been placed on dreams.

Fast forward to today, with sleep scientists now studying REM sleep in state-of-the-art laboratories with the use of electroencephalography (EEG), and we have gained marvellous insights about the functions and benefits of dreaming, namely emotional regulation.

Dreams and Emotional Regulation

WE NOW KNOW much more than we ever did about why we dream but remain in the dark about what our dreams mean. A lack of understanding for many equates to a lack of interest. In the modern era, dreams are too easily and often dismissed. Many people report never dreaming or say that if they do, they have no memory of the dream or the content. Several studies report that the higher the dream recall a person has, the more creative their thinking is. A study published in the *Journal of Creative Behavior* divided 125 participants into two groups after an initial baseline test on levels of creativity. The first group were asked to keep a dream log for 27 days, and the second were asked to record a memory from the previous day as vividly as possible. The researchers discovered that those who logged their dreams displayed higher levels of creativity at the end of the study and were less likely to fall into stereotypical or rigid thinking.[33]

Many indigenous people still practise rituals today that pay due diligence to the magical world of dreams. For example, Dreamtime refers to a spiritual belief held by the Aboriginal people in Australia that ancestral beings created the world; it is also an ongoing tradition practised through storytelling, song and dance and art. *Hatsuyume* is the Japanese word given to the first dream people have on 1 January, and it is said to predict your fortune for the new year. In Native American culture, the practice of 'dream incubation' involves setting an intention to dream about a particular topic or to bring clarity to an important decision.

On average, a good sleeper (like you are now) will spend 20 per cent–25 per cent of their 8-hour sleep in REM. So, even if you don't recall your dreams (and you are not taking medication that interferes with REM, such as sleeping tablets), you are dreaming. Being connected to your dreams brings you closer to them.

When we refer to having a dream, we don't necessarily mean one that we had while we were sleeping. The expression 'follow your dreams' suggests we find the courage it takes to pursue our goals while we are awake.

> **What is your deepest waking desire? What do you dream of being or doing? Do you cast off some of the goals you have as unrealistic and unattainable? Do you limit yourself?**

Could it be that your 'waking dreams' and desires remain unrealised because you are ignoring the messages within the dreams you have at night? Whatever you would like to manifest in your waking world, the fears that block you and the guidance you need are often released in your dreams while you sleep. Sleep scientist Matthew Walker's hypothesis is that 'dreams are not forgotten, merely inaccessible, and the impact they have on our waking selves is significant'.

Ignoring the remarkable insights that you glean from dreams is something you can change easily by taking just a few moments before you go to sleep and when you rise to connect more deeply to the hidden gems they provide. Your dreams are a window into your subconscious. When you begin to give them the attention they deserve, you will marvel at the impact they have on your understanding of yourself and the world around you.

In addition, recalling your dreams creates another positive association with sleep. You begin to genuinely look forward to the messages within your dreams and how you can harness their power to shape your life for the better. Each night when you go to sleep, a full production crew assembles to produce and direct a film for your viewing pleasure only. You are the main character and the film you are watching has been created to cleanse and regulate your emotions while also providing precise insights to help you to live your life with more clarity and meaning. The answers you seek to the challenges you face and the decisions you make are within your dreams.

Dream analysis is often met with scepticism and can be seen as superstitious. This is both unfortunate and understandable. As I mentioned, sleep science is now beginning to understand why we dream. Books that offer standardised dream interpretations tend to generalise what is highly subjective. For example, if you dream of your teeth falling out this means anxiety, insecurity, or a loss of power or control; that seems obvious. Understanding why *you* are anxious is much more beneficial. Dream interpretation is a highly personal thing that can only be done within the context of the individual and, indeed, by the person themselves.

YOU are the only person who can attempt to interpret your own dreams.

In the same way that you observe your mind during the day, you observe it at night, without judgement and with the intention of learning more about what makes you *you*. As you progress through your 90-minute sleep cycles, REM becomes longer in duration and more intense, so if, like me, you wake up in the morning either in the middle of or towards the end of a dream, you may feel slightly discombobulated for those first few moments. These moments are precious windows into your emotional world and it's important to consciously connect to them. Dr Rick Hanson, a psychologist with whom I trained in positive neuroplasticity, spoke of his Jungian therapist, who valued the importance of dream work and told him, 'When the unconscious realises that someone is listening, it starts to communicate.'

✦ ✦ ✦

Turning Subconscious Chaos Into Conscious Clarity

FOLLOW THESE STEPS to begin to understand your dreams.

In the morning when you wake, stay completely still for a few moments. Breathe deeply, have your journal close by and then write out whatever you can recall. Being as specific as you can, describe the events, the people and, most important, the feelings that were created in your dream. It doesn't matter if it makes no sense – write down as much as you can. If nothing comes at all, simply focus on how you feel in your body. Dreams fade fast, so the sooner you can do this, the better.

Last thing at night before you go to sleep, set the intention of remembering your dreams. Ryan Hurd, a dream and consciousness expert, suggests asking yourself the following four questions before you go to sleep:

✦ Was there anything that bothered me today?

✦ What was the most meaningful experience I had today?

✦ Did I have any insights or realisations today?

✦ What am I looking forward to tomorrow?

Asking yourself these questions primes your subconscious to make sense of your waking world and offer you solutions as you dream.

You may still feel that you are not aware of your dreams, but this will begin to shift as your sleep continues to improve. By consciously paying attention to dreams you are building a newfound awareness, curiosity and above all respect for the messages of your dreams.

✦ ✦ ✦

Nightmares and Night Terrors

IF YOU SUFFER from nightmares and/or night terrors, please don't despair. Remember Fionnuala's sleep story (p. 17). She stopped having nightmares and night terrors thanks to both her commitment and courage to address the underlying anxiety that was causing them.

A night terror is not technically a dream but an extreme fear reaction when you are transitioning from deep sleep into REM. Reactions include kicking, screaming, crying and a pounding heart. The cause of these dramatic disturbances can be exceptionally high levels of stress or post-traumatic stress disorder (PTSD).

The *Universal Etymological English Dictionary*, a popular reference text in the 1700s, defined nightmares as 'a disease when a man in his sleep supposes he has a great weight laying upon him'. It is quite accurate, as many people describe a heavy feeling in their chest after experiencing a nightmare, which is an extreme form of a bad dream.

As discombobulating as they are, occasional nightmares are normal and, in fact, necessary to help you to process stress and anxiety, especially if you are having a particularly challenging time in your life, such as the loss of a loved one, a divorce, financial pressure or even moving house.

The most prevalent time to experience nightmares is when you are a child aged three to six years old, as the young brain is desperately trying to make sense of the world. The young brain (as you learned earlier) is predominantly in the theta brainwave and therefore the imagination is more active. Between 50 per cent and 85 per cent of healthy adults report the occasional nightmare, and it is nothing to be concerned about. When I have one, I am grateful to my subconscious for helping me to process difficult emotions.

A nightmare disorder is when you fail to get sufficient sleep due to experiencing more than one nightmare a week. It is estimated that as many as 2 per cent to 8 per cent of people suffer from this.[34] If you are concerned that you may be in this cohort, please answer the following questions provided by the American Academy of Sleep Medicine:

✦ Do you often wake up from sleep due to a disturbing dream?

✦ Do these dreams evoke emotions of fear, anger, sadness or disgust?

✦ Are you alert and able to think clearly as soon as you wake up?

✦ Are you able to clearly recall the details of these dreams?

✦ Do these dreams often occur during the late portion of your sleep period, such as in the early morning part of your sleep?

✦ Do you have difficulty falling back to sleep after these dreams?

- Do you ever suffer from sleep paralysis (the phenomenon of not being able to move your body when you are going to sleep or waking up)? Recall Fionnuala (Week One) experienced this when her sleep was at its most dire.

If you answered yes to most of these questions, it is worth seeking further help from a professional therapist to deal with the underlying cause of your anxiety.

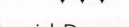

Lucid Dreaming

A LUCID DREAM is when the dreamer is aware that they are dreaming and is also able to control the dream. In other words, you become the director of your nightly movie, not just a spectator. For many years, scientific circles dismissed this phenomenon. Today science leaves no room for scepticism: lucid dreaming is a real occurrence. A meta-analysis study in 2016 looking at 50 years' worth of research found that 55 per cent of the population report having at least one lucid dream in their lifetime, 10 per cent–20 per cent say they have one a month and only 1 per cent report one per week.[35] Age also plays a factor, with more children and adolescents entering the state than adults.[36]

Stephen LaBerge, an American psychophysiologist (the branch of psychology that examines the influence of the mind on physical conditions, for example migraines caused by stress) is a pioneer in the field of lucid dreaming. LaBerge has conducted almost forty years of research into this area in his lab at Stanford University. His 2004 book *Lucid Dreaming: A Concise Guide to Awakening in Your Dreams and in Your Life* encourages the reader to learn how to consciously dream to increase creativity, build emotional resilience and create a positive impact on their waking world. In the late 1980s he conducted the first experiment to prove the validity of people's claims that they could control their dreams.[37] He did this by priming his subjects before they slept with a set of agreed eye movements – an 'ocular Morse code' – to communicate with. For example, three flicks to the left meant 'I am now lucid.'

In the same way that a person is paralysed in a normal REM state, the lucid dreamer has no way, apart from their eyes, to communicate to sleep scientists that they have now entered a lucid dreaming state. The prefrontal cortex (the part of your brain under your conscious control) is usually offline in a normal dream state, but in a lucid dream it is active in the same way as when you are awake. If you are interested in trying to induce a lucid dream, there is some new data from the University of Adelaide to support that it is challenging but possible. Out of a cohort of 47 people, 17 per cent were able to successfully induce a lucid dream.[38] Both of the following techniques require commitment and continued effort:

THE MILD (MNEMONIC INDUCTION OF LUCID DREAMS) METHOD

✦ Before you go to sleep, create a deliberate intention to remember as you dream that you are dreaming. Affirm, 'The next time I'm dreaming, I will remember that I'm dreaming.'

✦ If you wake up after a dream in the middle of the night, repeat the phrase again.

✦ Repeat this again and again as a mantra night after night.

THE REALITY TESTING METHOD

During the waking day, you begin to test reality, for example by touching a wall, or turning a light on and off. This illustrates you are awake according to the laws of physics. Keep doing this during your waking day until it becomes a habit. The desired outcome is that eventually you will begin to do this in your dreams, and when, for example, the light doesn't go on or off, you become aware that you are dreaming.

Why would you go to this effort? Curiosity would be for many a strong motive; however, it is worth keeping in mind both the benefits and disadvantages that are reported by lucid dreamers. The perks include increased emotional regulation and self-awareness, and fewer nightmares. The disadvantages include more fatigue and confusion over what is real and not.

Personally, I feel recording my dreams is both preferable and fascinating. I choose to let my subconscious roam where it will and then apply that curiosity to see insights in my daily life. One day I may try one of these methods, but for now, my conscious mind needs that time to go offline.

✦ ✦ ✦

Build your Sleep Well Habits

CONTINUE WITH THE habits you've formed in the previous weeks, I know it can seem like a lot, but you will already be doing some of these habits. The idea is that they are added incrementally and that you start to recognise which ones are most valuable to you. You have agency to choose what works best for you and to tweak each habit according to your own routine and schedule.

✦ Habit One: You go to sleep and wake up at roughly the same time every day.

✦ Habit Two: You have a 'blissful hour' bedtime routine.

✦ Habit Three: You move your body.

HABIT FOUR

Reduce Your Intake of Caffeine and Alcohol

All things in moderation, including moderation.

Attributed to SOCRATES

I LOVE THIS quote as it encapsulates the importance of remaining flexible with the eight sleep well habits. I don't want you to feel limited by them but liberated. There will be days and times where moderation needs a well-deserved break. Avoiding extremes in all forms, including, rather ironically, moderation, is healthy.

Having just explored the importance of dreaming for your emotional regulation, the habit for this week – 'Reduce your intake of caffeine and alcohol' – is one that will really boost your overall mood and ability to build emotional resilience. Both caffeine and alcohol are major disrupters to your REM sleep.

No caffeine after 12 p.m. and if you drink alcohol, do it in the early evening!

Let's tackle caffeine first. As Sat Bir pointed out in the interview above, you can mimic the effects of insomnia simply by consuming caffeine. It is an arousing stimulant that is designed to keep us awake and alert.

The average adult experiences a caffeine half-life of approximately five to six hours. This means that half of the caffeine you consume remains in your system for five to six hours after having that cup of coffee. Additionally, caffeine has a quarter-life of around ten to twelve hours, which is a long time and not something you would usually consider. If, for example, you have a cup of coffee at 2 p.m., at midnight a quarter of that caffeine might still be circulating in your brain.

The impact this caffeine has on your sleep quality is significant even if you are one of those people who has an espresso after dinner at 11 p.m. and falls asleep straight after. The research reveals that caffeine can reduce the amount of deep sleep, particularly stages three and four of non-REM sleep.[39] Consequently, upon waking up the next morning, you may not feel as restored or refreshed by your sleep. You may not recall struggling to fall asleep or waking up during the night and thus, you fail to make the connection. Subsequently, you find yourself reaching for two or three cups of coffee the next morning to feel wide awake due to what we call non-restorative sleep.

People's sensitivity to caffeine can vary greatly, but a simple rule is to minimise tea and coffee, with a maximum of three cups a day and no later than ten hours before you go to bed. Tea drinkers often don't make the connection between consuming tea later in the day and the impact it has on their sleep. There is, of course, less caffeine in tea, yet, depending on factors such as the type of tea, brewing time and water temperature, a 240 ml cup of brewed black tea contains about 40–70 milligrams (mg) of caffeine, while the same amount of brewed coffee typically contains around 95–165 mg of caffeine. In other words, a strong cup of tea is not significantly weaker than a weak cup of coffee. Green tea generally has a lower caffeine content, ranging from 20–45 mg per 240 ml cup.

What this Looks Like for Me

I drink tea and sometimes a coffee in the morning. I wait an hour after getting up before I have my first cup of caffeinated tea (this helps to prevent an afternoon slump). I usually have two, no more than three, caffeinated drinks a day. Green tea is a favourite. I switch to herbal teas after 12 p.m. and love a night-time cup of chamomile.

ALCOHOL

NOW FOR THE alcohol – stay with me, I promise it is worth it.

When you consume alcohol before bedtime (and, in particular, close to going to sleep), it interferes with the overall quality of your sleep. Many people use the sedative property of alcohol to knock themselves out quickly, and this does give the illusion of being beneficial. However, similar to a sleeping tablet, it is a false friend and actually causes significant disruption to your sleep. If a person is stressed, working hard, worried about a family member or an illness and has a racing mind before bed, we can understand why they would have a desire to numb their senses and reach oblivion quickly. Of course, this only serves to double the stress the next morning, rather than minimise it, as now the person has a hangover and/or depleted energy to deal with their issues.

Alcohol amplifies stress.

When you drink alcohol, even moderately, one of the reasons you do not feel refreshed the next day is that you have got roughly half the quality of sleep you would have done without any alcohol.[40] The Sleep Foundation, which is the leading source for evidence-based, medically reviewed sleep health information, states that:

- Low alcohol intake (less than two drinks for men and less than one for women) decreases sleep quality by 9.3 per cent.

- Moderate alcohol intake (two drinks for men and one drink for women) decreases the quality by 24 per cent.

- High alcohol consumption (more than two drinks for men and more than one for women), which by many people's standards may not seem high at all, decreases the benefits of sleep by 39.2 per cent.

A further detrimental effect alcohol has on your sleep is that it is a REM suppressant, and when you forgo your dreams you pay the price emotionally and mentally. A sleep spindle is a burst of electrical activity that rates ten to fifteen Hertz in frequency and is released during the transition into stage two REM sleep. Sleep spindles are integral to synaptic plasticity and play a significant role in memory consolidation.

Remember, we are not striving for perfection, but reducing your alcohol is going to help you to improve the quality of not only your sleep, but your life. The more present, patient and peaceful you are, the less you have the desire to drink alcohol in large quantities, if at all.

Waking up to full consciousness and reality means you have no desire to numb it.

If you do like to have a drink, then make sure it is at least four hours from your sleep time (not bedtime). This will give ample time for your body to metabolise the alcohol before the onset of sleep.[41] If you do drink too close to bedtime on occasion, drink lots of water and get back into your routine the next night.

What this Looks Like for Me

I drink alcohol, but very rarely. If I do have an occasional drink, it will be at aperitif time (6 p.m.) and something low in alcohol, like a beer or prosecco. I have seen first hand the destruction alcohol does to individuals and their families. I believe that culturally we have normalised what can be a very dangerous drug. If you suffer from anxiety or stress, drinking alcohol is the worst thing you can do for yourself.

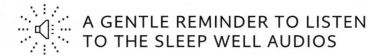

A GENTLE REMINDER TO LISTEN TO THE SLEEP WELL AUDIOS

You can access these audios for FREE with the passcode ISLEEPWELL on www.thepositivehabit.com.

Please remember to listen to the instructions for listening to guarantee maximum benefits.

MORNING MEDITATION

Please listen each morning to 'Start Your Day in Stillness – Intention-Setting Morning Meditation' to slow down your thoughts, before the day commences.

AFTERNOON OR EVENING REST RITUAL

Please listen to 'Seven-Minute Rest Ritual' each afternoon and/ or evening.

NIGHT-TIME HYPNOTHERAPY – WEEK FOUR: HABIT FOUR

This is the most important track to listen to. Each week there are new subconscious suggestions to help to reinforce the corresponding weekly habit and the following key insights.

To Get Back to Sleep if You Wake Up

You can listen to your night-time audio again, if necessary, but with time you will not need to do this. The Sleep Well Formula (Breathe + Imagine + Experience = Faith) which you are learning on a subconscious level every time you listen to your weekly audios will become automatic. Please also listen to the '4, 7, 8 Breathing' audio and train yourself to do this in the middle of the night should you awaken.

THE GOLDEN KEY INSIGHTS FROM WEEK FOUR: YOUR SLEEPING SELF

✦ For the first seven years of life, theta is our predominant brainwave state. These years are very formative in terms of conditioned beliefs. Theta is also present in adults in the onset of sleep, deep relaxation, creativity, enhanced learning, deep meditation and, in particular, hypnosis. Theta is a very malleable state for subconscious change.

✦ Sleep architecture is the term used to describe the sleep journey from beginning to end. Each cycle lasts roughly 90–120 minutes and the number of cycles you have can vary from four to six each night. Everyone will have a unique pattern, yet none of us can skip a stage. You want to ensure you have an 8-hour sleep opportunity each night.

✦ If you wake up in the middle of the night or early in the morning, please apply the Sleep Well Formula silently to yourself in your mind. The sooner you intervene before the conscious mind takes full control, the faster you will return to a deeper sleep.

- What is your deepest waking desire? What do you dream of being or doing? Do you cast off some of the goals you have as unrealistic and unattainable? Do you limit yourself? Could it be that your 'waking dreams' and desires remain unrealised because you are ignoring the messages in the dreams you have at night?

- A nightmare disorder is when you fail to get sufficient sleep due to experiencing more than one nightmare a week. It is estimated that as many as 2 per cent to 8 per cent of people suffer from this. If you are in this cohort please seek medical help.

- Habit Four is 'Reduce your intake of caffeine and alcohol'.

To maximise the benefits of this programme, I encourage you not to begin reading Week Five until you have listened to the 'Week Four: Habit Four' night-time audio for a minimum of seven nights in total.

Remember to keep building your habits and to introduce this week's one gently. It is important to take your time and remain patient with yourself. Your best is always good enough and your best is also likely to change on any given day. Please remember to acknowledge all progress with your habits and mindset, no matter how big or small.

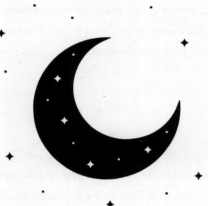

EMBRACE THE CHALLENGES

Believe in yourself and all that you are. Know that there is something inside you that is greater than any obstacle.

CHRISTIAN D. LARSON

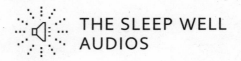

THE SLEEP WELL AUDIOS

All audios are available to download on www.thepositivehabit.com with the password ISLEEPWELL.

✦ Tonight, please start listening to 'Week Five: Habit Five' of your Sleep Well audios. Please listen to this audio for a minimum of seven nights. Please do not skip ahead to Week Six until you have listened for a full seven days.

✦ Please also continue to listen to your morning meditation and your rest ritual tracks each day.

✦ ✦ ✦

Measure Your Sleep

BEFORE YOU BEGIN Week Five of the Sleep Well Programme, please take a moment to rate your sleep. On a scale of 0 to 10, how well have you slept in the last week? (0 is 'terribly' and 10 is 'very well'.) Please use the image on the opposite page to mark where you feel you are on this scale.

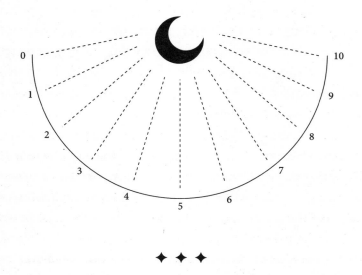

✦ ✦ ✦

Welcome to Week Five

CONGRATULATIONS, YOU ARE just over the halfway mark. Thank you so much for coming this far with me. Transforming your sleep takes time, as you know, and cannot be rushed. The Greeks have a saying, 'siga, siga', which translates as 'slowly, slowly'. I say this to myself often if I find I am heading towards overwhelm. Wherever you are on your sleep journey, you are exactly where you need to be. Be sure to use the Law of Least Effort (from Week One). Remember, sleep is not something you try to do, in the same way you don't try to make your heart beat – it just beats once you look after it. Keep listening to your audios and let them do all the heavy lifting on a subconscious level. Having said this, the Law of Least Effort is not the law of *no* effort: your conscious input and commitment to the process are also required. Your best is always good enough.

At this stage you are likely to be much more aware of the impact your personal sleep story had on your sleep and the thoughts and beliefs that you once held and that were holding you back. This programme is a new sleep chapter in your life, and each night you get the opportunity to begin again, a whole new night to rest, sleep and dream. Bedtime has become a time of the day to relish rather than dread.

Now that I (hopefully) have you feeling warm and positive, I do need to forewarn you that this week's topic is probably the toughest on our path so far. This is because I am going to cover the principal sleep challenges, and you may be navigating one or more of these right now; perhaps it is the reason you bought this book. Or perhaps, like many other people, you are no longer directly dealing with the challenge; however, your sleep may have never fully recovered from it. For example, maybe you had a baby who cried so much at night that even though your child is now a teenager, you still wake up fully during the night. Or perhaps you lost a loved one years ago and your sleep was very broken when you dealt with the shock, and even though you have come to terms (as much as you can) with the loss, the fragmented sleep pattern remains.

I would not be fulfilling my promise to you if I didn't cover these issues that are real and genuine concerns for so many. Embracing these challenges now means that you will be in a prime state to move forward with the remaining three weeks, which cover the sleep strengths of presence, patience and peace. I promise you it is worth the effort and the reward is a sustainable shift in your relationship with sleep. You will enter into a lifelong love affair with sleep and it will see you through your toughest times. It will keep you healthy and wise and it will always bring out your brightest, lightest self.

With sleep by your side, no issue is insurmountable and you have the emotional resilience you need to flourish in the world.

Each of the following challenges is worthy of a book in its own right. I am providing a brief overview of the main obstacles, including insomnia and its criteria, to help you seek further help if necessary. It is important that context is provided for those of you who may be navigating one or more of these challenges right now, for example hot flushes at night, chronic pain or having a young baby.

Whatever YOUR situation is, continue to apply the Sleep Well Formula (Breathe + Imagine + Experience = Faith) and you will improve the effectiveness of your sleep. It won't be perfect, but it will most certainly be better. Remember the two-arrow parable: many situations are out of your control, but your response is always within your grasp.

✦ ✦ ✦

Insomnia

INSOMNIA IS A serious clinical disorder for people who have an overactive sympathetic nervous system; this means that their stress response never turns off and they remain in a state of high alert during the night. This heightened state has damaging biological consequences, including inflammation which can trigger the onset of various non-communicable diseases. A racing heart and raised metabolic rate increase the core body temperature, making sleep impossible. In addition, cortisol levels are generally excessive due to the increased levels of anxiety.[42]

The American Academy of Sleep Medicine classifies insomnia as a 'persistent difficulty with sleep initiation, duration, consolidation or quality'.[43]

About ten per cent of the world's population will be clinically diagnosed with insomnia and one out of every two people will suffer from it at some stage in their life. Clinicians further divide insomnia into two categories based on two criteria. The first is the duration, how long it has been going on; and the second is the cause. Primary insomnia is a condition on its own and secondary insomnia is caused by another condition, such as chronic pain.

Insomnia is a classic vicious cycle: a person has a bout of bad nights' sleep and somnophobia (sleep anxiety) kicks in, and the build-up of pressure before going to bed intensifies. They feel anxious because they can't sleep, and their anxiety prevents them from falling asleep. So, which comes first? This is a bidirectional condition; in other words, one problem feeds into the other.

In my clinical experience, a two-pronged approach is most effective: first of all getting to the roots of the anxiety and then addressing it with lifestyle intervention. This method is echoed in this book for you as we continue to work on both a psychological and a physiological level. Your weekly habits are all proven lifestyle interventions that can have a hugely positive impact on the overall quality of your sleep.

THE 30/30/3 RULE

The 30/30/3 rule of thumb is a method many clinicians worldwide use to determine whether a person has an insomnia disorder. The 30/30/3 rule is:

- It takes you at least 30 minutes to fall asleep.

- It takes you 30 minutes or more to go back to sleep if you wake in the middle of the night.

- This is happening at least 3 nights a week for three consecutive months.

THE THREE PS MODEL

An insomnia disorder usually commences from what is called, by sleep scientists, the '3 Ps model'.

Predisposition

Certain types of genes can play a role in your chances of developing the condition. For example, if one of your parents suffers from it, heritability rates can be as high as 28 per cent–45 per cent.[44] Please remember, though, that like many hereditary conditions, whether it is a sleep disorder or heart disease, your lifestyle can make the difference between those genes being expressed or remaining dormant.

For example, a person may inherit pre-diabetic type two genes that make them more likely to suffer from the condition, but by being aware of this and making sensible lifestyle choices they will greatly lower their risk of activating these genes.[45] The same is true of insomnia. Often, the genes need to be flicked into action by, for example, a secondary contributing factor. If one or both of your parents suffer from insomnia, please don't adopt a fatalistic view. You can be the person who breaks the genetic chain.

Precipitation

An external trigger in a person's life causes an insomniac episode, for example a bereavement, a divorce or chronic stress at work. Please note, it is normal to suffer from poorer quality sleep during periods of increased stress and trauma. Once the stress has passed, though, the person remains on high alert and their parasympathetic nervous system remains switched off.

Perpetuating Factors

An ongoing condition that is causing insomnia, for example, alcohol or drug addiction, or living in a situation where you do not feel safe, for example an abusive relationship or in a war zone.

Remember the 'complaining good sleepers' we discussed in Week Two? Another factor that can prolong insomnia is what clinicians call 'sleep state misperception' or 'paradoxical insomnia'; this is when a person will severely underestimate the quality of their sleep.[46] Subjectively, the insomniac will measure it as very bad, but when measured objectively in a sleep lab it is significantly better than the person estimated. The prevalence of people who suffer with this form of insomnia ranges from 9.2% to 56%.[47] In a sleep lab, results will show that people who believe that they did not sleep a wink had, in fact, a full night's sleep. In the past, people with this condition were dismissed; however, this mismatch has a genuine impact on an individual and sleep doctors now, thankfully, take this condition seriously.

The single most damaging side effect of insomnia, whatever the form or cause, is the psychological distress it causes. When it comes to anxiety and sleep, it is often a case of mutual causality. The higher levels of cortisol caused by the anxiety will affect your sleep and the lack of sleep will leave you feeling on edge and vulnerable. One example of this was seen globally during the Covid-19 pandemic. Researchers at the University of Southampton conducted a systematic review and meta-analysis of 42 studies that included over 80,000 participants from around the world, and they found that the rise in anxiety over the pandemic caused sleep disturbances, with each condition exacerbating the other.[48]

✦ ✦ ✦

Sleep Deprivation and the Scary Sleep Science

SLEEP DEPRIVATION HAS for centuries been used as a form of torture and as a means to weaken a person's resolve when being interrogated. So much so that it was once called an 'enhanced interrogation technique'. It is an act of extreme cruelty and the side effects on an individual are serious, leading to hallucinations, psychosis and symptoms similar to schizophrenia. A person will agree to almost anything to be allowed to sleep.

Side effects of insomnia during the day include a general exhaustion that doesn't lift, constant sleepiness, never feeling refreshed, difficulty focusing, forgetfulness, irritability, lack of emotional regulation, hypersensitivity, conflicts in relationships (personal and at work), inability to problem-solve, catastrophising, impaired academic performance, hyperactivity, depression, lack of motivation and a higher risk of driving errors or household accidents. It is not a pretty list and not one I want for you, dear reader.

I did promise you this is not a sleep book with scary sleep science, so please take a moment and consider that the opposite of this list is what we are cultivating now as you change your relationship with sleep: feeling revitalised when you wake, increased energy during the day, high levels of concentration, responding and not reacting emotionally, feeling calm, behaving considerately, being mindful, alert, forgiving and kind, harmony in your relationships, success at work, identifying solutions easily after a good night's sleep, feeling optimistic and motivated overall, better motor skills and balance.

This is all yours now.

A chronic lack of sleep is a serious issue, and it cannot be ignored. I am not a medical doctor and diagnosing insomnia disorder requires consulting a qualified doctor who specialises in sleep medicine. **If you believe you are suffering from insomnia, please contact a doctor while you continue this eight-week course.**

✦ ✦ ✦

Night-Shift Work

NIGHT WORKERS CAN feel like they are the living dead. The day is night and vice versa. The challenges they face are many, including a disrupted circadian clock, increased fatigue due to disturbed sleep, increased health risks and feeling disconnected from family and friends. Many essential services must operate 24 hours a day and staff are required to work nights. These people deserve more recognition for their contribution to society and also more help to optimise their sleep. This is a book in itself waiting to be written. If you are a night shift worker, thank you for all you do, whether that is in health care, a call centre or cleaning the streets. What you do is valuable, and you deserve the best help you can get to improve your sleep.

Fortunately, several effective tools can help improve your sleep quality and overall well-being. First and foremost, establishing a consistent sleep routine, even on days off, can anchor the body's internal clock and promote better sleep. You need to turn day into night, and your light exposure is the most effective way to do this. Create a conducive sleep environment by using blackout curtains, earplugs or white noise machines during daytime sleep. If you are returning from work while it is getting light, wear shades to keep out as much light as possible.

Incorporating short naps strategically during long shifts can provide a quick energy boost without disrupting sleep patterns. Communicating with employers and colleagues about the importance of sleep and seeking flexible scheduling options when possible is also a good idea.

You can and should still apply all the habits in the course; however, the single most effective difference is that your light exposure is in reverse. When you get home, start your unwinding routine 60 minutes before sleep. The impact of night work on sleep is an area that needs a lot of attention as more and more people are required to work at night. Statistics vary globally on the number of people who have to work the night shift, also known as 'the graveyard shift'. In the US it is about 7.4 per cent of the working population with a higher number of this percentage being male and non-white. In Europe the figures are higher and the latest EU Labour Force survey, covering 28 countries, indicates that 16.7 per cent of employed men and 9.4 per cent of employed women worked night shifts in 2018.[49]

There is evidence to suggest that some people can adapt and get used to working night shifts over time. This process is often referred to as 'shift work adaptation' or 'circadian adaptation.' The human body has a remarkable ability to adjust its internal circadian rhythm to align with new sleep–wake schedules, including night shifts. If you are not one of these people (bearing in mind that age, genetics and lifestyle factors all impact on your likelihood of adapting), please do consider talking to your management about coming off night shifts or looking for a new job entirely. Your sleep and your life have to come first.

Flatlining Cortisol Levels

DIURNAL CORTISOL SLOPES refer to the release of cortisol over the course of 24 hours. A healthy release of cortisol spikes shortly after awakening and then slowly decreases as the day goes on, with low levels at night allowing for a smooth transition to sleep.

A flatlining curve is both a cause and an effect for some people with poor sleep and those who live in a consistent state of stress. If you suffer from flatlining cortisol levels it means that you will struggle to regulate your release of cortisol levels at the appropriate times during the day. Flatlining can also be caused by certain medications and adrenal insufficiency. Adrenal insufficiency is a medical condition in which the adrenal glands (located on top of the kidneys) are not producing enough of certain hormones, in particular cortisol.

If you feel that your cortisol curve is out of balance, it could be worth asking your doctor for either a blood or urine test. There are also saliva tests that will measure cortisol levels at various times of the day to give you a more detailed analysis. There have been various studies to indicate that practising formal meditation will help to balance the diurnal cortisol rhythm.[50] With this and the other protocols in the Sleep Well Programme, you are no longer at the mercy of external stressors, but through loving awareness, you intervene and return your system to balance. When you feel balanced, you sleep.

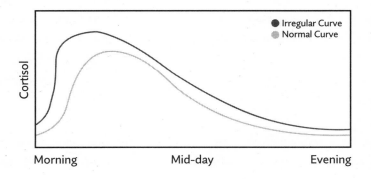

‣ ‣ ‣

Restless Legs Syndrome (RLS)

RLS IS A neurological disorder characterised by uncomfortable sensations in the legs, often accompanied by an irresistible urge to move them. It can lead to difficulty falling asleep and disrupted sleep throughout the night. Soaking in a warm bath before bed and massaging the legs can relax the muscles. Applying warm or cool packs may lessen limb sensations.

Challenges for Women

RESEARCH INDICATES THAT women are 40 per cent more likely to suffer from insomnia than men; unsurprisingly, women are also twice as likely to suffer from anxiety.[51] (Keep in mind that when it comes to mental health and gender statistics it is hard to get accurate data, as many men do not report their symptoms.) As you know, a lack of sufficient sleep creates anxiety and anxiety creates insufficient sleep. This is why this book is designed to tackle anxiety and sleep on both a biological and a psychological level.

Each stage of a woman's life comes with unique challenges when it comes to sleep, from adolescence to menopause and through to old age.[52] Sleep disruptions are often due to a fluctuation in hormones interrupting sleeping patterns. A young girl starting her period will have a huge influx of oestrogen and a pregnant woman will have an increase in progesterone; these significant shifts can cause broken sleep.

In addition to these issues, one study published in the *Journal of Sleep* by a research team led by Dr Jim Horne, a sleep expert at Loughborough University, indicated that women generally need around twenty minutes' more sleep than men. The reasons for this are:

✦ Women tend to have busier schedules and multitask

✦ Hormonal changes

- ✦ Not enough rest in the daytime

- ✦ The neurochemistry in the female brain is wired to optimise analytical thinking.[53]

If you are female, looking at the list above will help you to identify areas that can be improved. For example, you can begin to take more rest, adopt a healthy lifestyle to help regulate and balance your hormones and practise meditation to slow down the impulse to multitask.

MENOPAUSE

For many women, the most disruptive period is perimenopause and menopause. Sleep disorders affect 39 per cent to 47 per cent of perimenopausal women and 35 per cent to 60 per cent of postmenopausal women.[54] The most common complaints are hot flushes, night sweats and anxiety. I was 44 when I first experienced the symptoms of perimenopause, and similar to many women, I was at a loss about what to do. I went to see a GP who specialised in the area, and she informed me of the benefits of hormone replacement therapy (HRT), which I immediately dismissed, despite having both osteoporosis and heart disease in my family. I believed taking it was a weakness.

I needed to navigate on my own through my mindset and lifestyle. A few months later I was back with the same doctor. The night sweats were so intense, and my sleep was beyond broken. I felt as vulnerable and anxious as when I was a teenager and knew I couldn't do it alone. Taking HRT was one of the best decisions I've made. It is not a panacea, and personally I believe it is only effective in conjunction with a very healthy lifestyle and a positive mindset.

I am gratefully sailing through a phase in my life that had the potential to cause chaos physically and emotionally. HRT is not for everyone. You need to make the choice that is correct for you and with professional medical supervision, taking into account your family history. There are alternatives for those who need it that are very helpful, so please don't suffer unnecessarily.

Male Challenges

MEN MAY NOT suffer from the rollercoaster of hormonal changes in the same way as women do, but they have their own set of issues to contend with. It is worth noting that this list is not exhaustive and many women also suffer from many of these challenges.

SLEEP APNOEA

Sleep apnoea is a sleep disorder characterised by repeated pauses in breathing during sleep.[55] It is two to three times more common in men, especially in middle-aged and older men. Obstructive sleep apnoea (OSA) is the more common form. It occurs when throat muscles relax and block the flow of air into the lungs; it is also accompanied by loud snoring. Central sleep apnoea (CSA) is when the brain fails to send the appropriate signals to the muscles responsible for breathing. The good news is that lifestyle changes, weight loss and the use of a continuous positive airway pressure (CPAP) device or even surgical intervention can ameliorate the condition considerably.

PROSTATE-RELATED ISSUES

Prostate-related issues can have an impact on older men's sleep. The prostate is a small gland located below the bladder and in front of the rectum. As men age, the prostate may undergo changes that can affect urinary function and, in turn, disrupt sleep. It's important to discuss any concerns you have about your prostate with a healthcare provider. Limiting fluid intake before bed is always a good idea, but even more so in this instance. Both caffeine and alcohol can act as diuretics and are also best avoided. In some cases, medications or medical procedures may be recommended to address prostate-related issues.

SUPPRESSED EMOTIONS AND DEPRESSION

The latest data we have on death by suicide from the Central Statistics Office is from 2019. In that year, there were 524 deaths from suicide in Ireland. Of those deaths, 408 were males.[56] Globally, the rate of suicide mortality in 2019 was 9/100,000 for both sexes together (12.6 in males versus 5.4 in females).[57] These sad and startling statistics are too stark to ignore. The unfortunate phrase 'man up' is indicative of a culture of toxic masculinity. Patriarchal conditioning begins at a very young age: at five or six, boys learn it is not OK to express emotion. For example, if a girl falls in the playground and cries, it is totally acceptable, but if a boy does the same, he is told to be strong. The boy quickly learns that in order to survive he needs to suppress his emotions and that showing them is a sign of weakness.

The Mayo Clinic states that men suffering from depression may display the following symptoms: feeling sad, hopeless or empty, extreme exhaustion, difficulty sleeping and/or sleeping too much, and no longer getting pleasure from activities they usually enjoy.[58] While these symptoms can also be seen in depressed women, men tend to also show signs of escapist behaviour, such as spending a lot of time at work or on sports. They also frequently have physical symptoms, such as headaches, digestive problems and pain, and display problems with alcohol or drug use and controlling, violent or abusive behaviour, irritability or inappropriate anger and risky behaviour, such as reckless driving.

If you suspect you are suffering from depression, regardless of the gender you identify with, please seek help from a qualified therapist and also speak to your GP. The stigma related to mental health issues has come a long way, but many men continue to suffer in silence and never seek the help they deserve.

✦ ✦ ✦

Relationship Issues

SOME COUPLES WHO try everything and still find they can't sleep together may eventually decide to sleep in separate rooms. The stigma around this needs to be removed. It doesn't mean the end of the relationship or of intimacy; often it is the opposite, and improved energy can lead to an increased sex drive. Another less dramatic option is to consider single beds that are together but have their own mattresses and duvets. You are far less likely to disturb your partner and you are together but also enjoying the comfort of your own space.

✦ ✦ ✦

Snoring

SNORING IS A lose–lose situation for both the snorer and the partner lying beside them.[59] The level of disruption it causes is not to be ignored. Constant interruptions to your sleep, as you know, have an impact on your overall sleep quality and will cause both parties to wake up less than refreshed and with their moods out of balance.

In truth, most of us snore sometimes, but it becomes an issue when it is chronic and loud. Being woken up nightly by a partner you love can put serious pressure on a relationship: the person who is constantly woken feels frustrated and the person snoring can feel guilty for causing the other to suffer. Like I said, a lose–lose. Sleep must come first so that both you and the relationship survive.

On a practical level, you can wear earplugs – they really do help! You can also try taping the mouth of the snorer. This sounds extreme, but James Nestor, author of *Breath: The New Science of a Lost Art*, swears by this as it helps to retrain you to breathe through your nose at night and prevents mouth-breathing and snoring. Sleeping on your side, avoiding alcohol and raising the head of your bed all help also. Becoming a deeper sleeper (if your partner is snoring) is the most effective solution – it has worked for me. I now rarely hear my husband snore after years of being disturbed. I do still wear earplugs, though!

Parenthood

IT'S 15 YEARS since my son was a baby, but I can still recall the fog of doing the night shifts of feeding and soothing him back to sleep at unearthly hours in the night and early morning. If you have had children or, much more important, currently have a baby or young children, you know exactly what I am talking about. The mixed feelings of both love and frustration melting into one another through blurry eyes and bottles. The sleep wars that often rage between partners (if you are fortunate enough to have a co-pilot) on the very rocky road of parenting a baby.

There is a lot of sleep literature on how to establish a sleeping routine for babies and it is always the first question young parents are asked: 'Are *they* sleeping yet?' The question that is not asked is 'Are *you* sleeping?' The assumption is that if the baby is not sleeping, then neither are the parents. However, one of the best things I did was to take sleep when I could. I napped during the day when Luca (my son) was asleep, and I took it in turns with my husband to work shifts so that we both got as much sleep as we could (I know this option is not available to all). Prioritising *your* sleep as a parent is (as you will read shortly in the next sleep story, by neuroscientist Dr Sarah McKay) essential to navigate the emotional terrain of being a new parent. The better-slept you are, the calmer you are. And the calmer you are, the sooner your baby will settle into a routine. It is not selfish, it is survival. You are also leading by example and teaching your young kids that sleep matters for both adults and children.

✦ ✦ ✦

Resistance

IN MY CLINICAL experience, it is normal about halfway through a person's journey for some resistance to arise, especially after a tough session that deals directly with a prolonged challenge they face, like sleep issues! Perhaps you might feel this also. (If not, wonderful, feel free to ignore me.) If you do feel any frustration, rest assured this is a normal and healthy response when you are making any significant changes in your lifestyle and mindset. To help you with this, can you bring to mind the image of your best-slept self and remind yourself of all the progress you have made so far? I intentionally waited to introduce the sleep challenges until now as I knew you would be ready to embrace them having had four weeks of improved sleep. When you sleep well you are in a position of strength to manage any setback that comes your way in life and sleep!

The sleep contract we signed remains at the heart of our continued work. Here is a gentle reminder of our commitment to one another.

> *I, Fiona Brennan, am committed to helping you to sleep peacefully to the best of my ability. The tools and insights shared in this book are based on up-to-date science and my wealth of clinical experience.*

Signed *Fiona Brennan*

> *I, ...,*
> *am committed to following the programme to the best of my ability and devoting myself to the love of sleep. I will be kind to myself. If I miss one night of the eight-week programme, I will simply start again the next.*

We keep going, night by night and breath by breath.

A Story of Prioritising:
Dr Sarah McKay

I FIRST MET Dr Sarah McKay when I interviewed her for my webcast series, 'Building Emotional Resilience'. As she spoke, I couldn't help but notice how many references she made to sleep and in particular her own positive relationship with it. Dr Sarah McKay is an Oxford-educated neuroscientist and the founder of the Neuroscience Academy. She is from New Zealand and lives in Sydney with her Irish husband and two teenage boys.

Sarah specialises in translating brain science research into simple, actionable strategies for peak performance, creativity, health and well-being. Sarah is incredibly sleep focused and designs her life around ensuring she is getting both the quality and quantity of sleep that she knows (on a personal and professional basis) she needs. She put it at the centre of her family's life when her two sons were born, and again now in her late forties, she is also ensuring that she gets the best sleep she possibly can. Both of these are times in many parents' and women's lives that they are sleep deprived. As you will see, Sarah sets the 'sleep bar' high; however, as I have said before, sleep is not a competition. You are finding your own way and I share this story to inspire you: no matter what stage of life you are in, you can optimise your sleep to be the best it can within the confines of your current life situation.

✦ ✦ ✦

I grew up in a house with a mum saying her favourite time of day was going to bed. Sleep was prioritised in my family. The bedtime routine was very calm, orderly and organised. It didn't feel strict, it just felt normal, we didn't question it. We would have a bath, read a story and go to sleep. I remember being at school and other kids would talk about TV programmes that I knew would have been on after I was in bed. It's a mindset that has been passed down the generations.

When I was a teenager and in my early twenties, I'd rather have been out at the pub or off to a rave. But when you're young, you don't get hangovers! Even then, though, I still remember during my final year of high school I'd be reading late, because I always read when I go to bed. My mum or dad would come in and gently suggest that I turn the light off. There was always an emphasis on sleep. I think it came from my mum's side, because all my aunts and cousins were the same – we would go on holiday, and we would all be in bed early.

At school, I was an overachiever and a classic perfectionist, and I ended up having a massive panic attack in my biology exam in my final year exams, but I don't remember my sleep being affected. However, I did find Covid super stressful with having the kids home from school and all the uncertainty. I was super stressed then, but I still slept really well. I do, however, remember waking up in the mornings, especially in March 2020, and feeling that panic rushing in.

My sleep is at its best now, which is rare for a woman in her forties. It's never not been great, but since I've been consciously aware of the neuroscience of sleep, I know how good it is. My boys are 13 and 15, so definitely within the last decade, as I've come out the other side of night-time wakings with kids, my sleep has got better and better.

I navigated the baby years by marrying well. My husband is a compliant man, and I was blessed with pretty straightforward babies. They weren't the kind of babies that cried all night long. I didn't have breastfeeding issues, so my husband was on duty from, say, 6 p.m. till midnight, and that meant I'd go to bed really early, by 7.30 p.m., and our baby would go down for the night. I implemented quite a day–night-time routine with my little boy from the beginning, and so my husband, Geoff, would 'be on' until midnight and had his one-on-one bonding time. I prioritised sleep before midnight and made sure I got 3–4 hours of deep restorative sleep. I had no qualms about heading off to bed at 7.30 p.m. or earlier. I was still tired but nowhere near as tired as I would have been if I had had a baby who didn't sleep or a husband who didn't help – like I said, I made sure to marry well! Sleep was and is a priority.

I am a big believer, especially with babies, that sleep begets sleep. If they are well rested and nap and sleep during the day, they'll be calm and sleep at night. I was always diligent about routines because I wanted my sleep to be protected. The two boys are both good sleepers today. My husband and I were a tag team and it worked.

I always get the whole morning sunlight that Andrew Huberman talks about [you will read about this in this week's habit]. I'm awake most mornings by six because we're very fortunate to have this lovely house that gets the morning sun and as soon as the horizon starts to lighten, I will wake up naturally.

Also, I am a strategic napper, so I don't just go, 'Oh I'm tired,' and fall asleep for three hours in the afternoon. I am very particular about how I nap. I would never nap for longer than half an hour and as early as I can after lunch. I probably nap five days out of seven. I have talked to loads of other people who have a specific napping routine, and they all sleep well at night as well. I call them strategic nappers.

I have a really strong positive sleep association, a strong psychological love and enjoyment of sleep. I wallow around in the pleasure of it and all the positive benefits that come from letting go and having a nap in the afternoon. Now the boys are older I actually lock the bedroom, but then the dog tries to sneak in – he's the disruptor in the family now! A few weeks ago, I was in the city, and I did all these morning interviews for my new book, and I had grabbed something to eat and was about to go home and then the television network rang and they said, 'Can you come into do a TV slot at four?' and it was about 1.30 p.m. and so my husband, Geoff, had driven into the city. So, I called him, and I said, 'Can I sleep in your car?'

> **A nap knocks off my rough emotional edges. It
> makes me feel more emotionally regulated.**

I would very rarely schedule something workwise in the evenings after dinner; that is my wind-down time. If I do have an evening presentation where I'm really 'on', I will find it harder to wind down after. I always have a shower before bed and I always, always read, even if I'm going to bed at 2 a.m. I never read non-fiction, and I'll read for half an hour and then I'm just like, 'I'm gonna fall asleep.' I'll usually put earplugs in, especially if Geoff's not in bed yet, and then I'm just asleep.

If for some reason I can't get to sleep, then I do something called cognitive reshuffling. This is where you choose a theme, say Olympic sports, and you find a sport starting with A and then B and so on. So instead of going into a default rumination mode or entertaining whatever drama you have in your imagination, you switch off. This has been shown to help people fall asleep. Very rarely would I get past F. It's usually when I am out of my routine that I need to use it.

I do break my routine sometimes to go out, to see a show, to have a few drinks. However, I won't break it just for anything, for a TV show, for example. It is very rare that something disrupts my sleep. My husband is like, 'You know nothing gets in the way of Sarah and her bed.' He always jokes that when I get into bed, the barriers go up and even the dog doesn't come near me.

The only times my sleep is disrupted now is if I drink alcohol, I get anxiety, or if I'm in a new environment, like a hotel. If I have one drink that is fine, but if I have three or four glasses, I really notice it. If I am sleeping somewhere new, for example I have to go to Melbourne for a talk, I am more alert. If I have earplugs, though, I am usually fine. I always travel with earplugs. If I have a big talk or presentation and I am at home, it doesn't make a difference to my sleep. It's just in new locations that I am super vigilant.

I'm protecting my sleep at all costs. It feels like the rest of the world is catching up on the significance of sleep on the brain for memory consolidation and emotional regulation. I am so glad that we did what we did with the boys when they were little. I was so protective of the family's health and my moods. We had no family support, so we did what we did to keep ourselves together in the best way. I knew sleep was the foundation for us and the kids and it still is.

✦ ✦ ✦

Build Your Sleep Well Habits

REMEMBER TO KEEP going with previous habits as you introduce a new one each week. See if you can stack any of the existing habits with the new ones – for example, you go for a run in the mid-morning before you have your last cup of caffeine for the day.

✦ Habit One: You go to sleep and wake up at roughly the same time every day.

✦ Habit Two: You have a 'blissful hour' bedtime routine.

✦ Habit Three: You move your body.

✦ Habit Four: You reduce your alcohol and caffeine intake.

HABIT FIVE

Optimise Your Light and Temperature Exposure

I am going to give my gratitude to the sun and to everything and everyone because I am still alive. One more day to be myself.

MIGUEL RUIZ, *THE FOUR AGREEMENTS: A PRACTICAL GUIDE TO PERSONAL FREEDOM*

WE KNOW THE sun as the giver of life, and it is also the provider of sleep. As Sarah McKay mentioned in her story above, she makes early morning light viewing a priority. Thanks to the work of Professor Andrew Huberman, the habit of early morning light exposure has become more widely practised.

In 1879, Thomas Edison and his team invented the light bulb. It seemed like a miracle as night was turned into day. Artificial light became widespread in the 1900s, and with it, sleep issues increased. All these extra hours of light increased productivity and certainly benefited the pockets of the tycoons of the industrial era.[60] The introduction of shift work now meant there was no dead time on the production line, yet the lives of people who worked in these industries were shortened. There was a rapid increase in health problems, including sleep disturbances, fatigue, gastrointestinal disorders, cardiovascular disease and metabolic disorders.

The connection between light and sleep interruption was not noticed at first. It was only in the 1950s and 1960s that it became an area of research.[61] One of the earliest studies in the area was conducted by scientists at the Institute of Mental Health, and published in the *American Journal of Science*. The researchers exposed participants to various levels of light at night and discovered that more light exposure at night meant less sleep.

Choosing to maximise and minimise your light exposure depending on the time of day is a powerful, practical and essential protocol that you need to implement immediately.

The Master Clock

The circadian rhythm is the body's internal 24-hour clock that regulates the sleep–wake cycle, the release of hormones, body temperature and other physiological issues. Each of these rhythms/ clocks is controlled by one 'master clock' in the brain.[62] The master clock is a group of cells in the brain called the suprachiasmatic nucleus (SCN), which is located in the hypothalamus. Light exposure is the prime means of setting this clock and establishing a healthy sleep cycle, hence also why the previous habit of going to bed and rising at the same time is so imperative.

In short, you want to get as much light as possible, as early in the day as you can, and then start to minimise it towards your bedtime. Like many of the best things in life, it is so painfully simple and often ignored. People will go to any lengths, including taking harmful medication, rather than stepping out into their garden or balcony as soon as they can after rising. If you want to sleep better, this habit is non-negotiable.

To practise this simple and highly effective habit, please ensure you hit these times.

View Direct Morning Light as Early as Possible After Rising

Go outside within 30–60 minutes of waking and soak in as much light as you can. If you wake up before the sun is up and you want to be awake, turn on artificial lights and then go outside as soon as the sun rises. On a very bright morning with no clouds, 10 minutes is sufficient; on cloudy days, 20 minutes; and on a very overcast day, 30–60 minutes is needed. Supplement this with as much artificial light as you can when indoors. (Clearly, don't look directly at the sun or you will burn your eyes. Do not wear sunglasses (eyeglasses and contacts are fine) or a wide-brimmed hat – but do wear sunscreen!)

Ideally, depending on the season, where you live on the planet and the time you have to get up for work, go outdoors as soon as you can around sunrise. The sunrise has a higher level of blue light.[63]

This blue light is the most effective at communicating with your master clock to release melatonin at the appropriate time in the evening and hence helping you glide to sleep. If, like many of us in the modern world, you cannot view the sunrise, then aim for 20–30 minutes outdoors as soon as you can after rising.[64]

Bright Light Therapy

If this is not possible because of long, dark winter mornings and/or your schedule, you need to use bright light therapy. In order to benefit from bright light therapy, the light needs to have a minimum of 10,000 lux, and the type that emits blue light is superior. The same amount of time, 30 minutes, is sufficient. You can easily purchase a device that emits bright white or blue light in the form of a box, a lamp or even glasses.

Nothing, however, is as strong as natural light, which can measure anywhere between 10,000 and 100,000 lux depending on cloud coverage. So, if the season is on your side – get outside. Go for a walk, or have breakfast in your garden or on your balcony if you have one.

If you use an alarm clock to wake up, switch to a sunrise alarm that emulates the natural sunrise. Waking with light rather than to the jarring sound of an alarm bell serves two purposes: you wake up peacefully and you are immediately exposed to maximum light.

Get Outside Again in the Evening and, if Possible, Watch the Sunset

As the evening progresses, start to minimise light exposure and avoid overhead lighting. Make sure the light in your bathroom when you brush your teeth is not too bright. Come off all screens 60 minutes before going to sleep. When you expose yourself to artificial light, and in particular the blue light from screens, before sleep, you delay the release of melatonin, the hormone that aids the onset of sleep. If you wake up in the night and need to go to the bathroom, only use as much artificial lighting as is necessary for you to move about safely. Candlelight (I find the fake ones effective) and moonlight are fine.

What this Looks Like for Me

In the lighter half of the year, I get up and get outside, before I shower or eat breakfast, for a gentle run, walk, yoga and/or meditation. In the evening, I get outside again at roughly the time the sun is setting and then I start to minimise bright lights. In the winter, I use light therapy to wake me up: I switch on all overhead lights and then get outside as soon as my schedule allows. I have also been known to wear shades travelling through airports after 10 p.m., not for egoic reasons but because I know it will help me to sleep. This habit has truly transformed and deepened the quality of my sleep. I notice the difference on the rare occasions I miss the morning light for a few days or have too much light exposure towards bedtime.

Drop the Temperature in Your Bedroom by 3 Degrees

The temperature of your body dictates how quickly you get to sleep and stay there. Have you ever noticed that you feel colder when you are tired? This is because the body's core temperature tends to drop slightly in the evening and reach its lowest point during the early morning hours. A cooler sleeping environment helps facilitate this temperature drop, signalling to the body that it's time to sleep.

Similar to light and food, start to control your temperature as soon as you rise. Follow these simple steps to utilise temperature as a tool to give you energy in the morning and to help you stay asleep all night long.

- When you get up in the morning, switch your shower to cold for a minimum of one minute and a maximum of three minutes, and you will start the day with lots of energy, feeling full of life. Paradoxically, cold water exposure increases your core body temperature.

- At the end of the day, a hot bath or shower heats up your body, and again ironically, your body temperature will then drop, which will make sleep easier.

- Make your bedroom very cool. Turn off any heating in this room at least 60 minutes before sleep time. The temperature in your bedroom probably needs to drop by at least three degrees and be around 16 degrees Celsius. Layers are best on the bed to ensure you are not cold but can throw off extra blankets if you wake up too hot. Open a window, even in winter, ever so slightly. The fresh air will improve air quality and ventilation. In the summer months in a very hot climate, turn on the air conditioning 60 minutes before you want to go to sleep. If you don't have air conditioning, bring a damp and cold face cloth to bed and put this on your forehead to help keep you cool. A water spray beside the bed can also be helpful.

Dropping your core body temperature by 1–3 degrees is not just important before sleep, it is essential to help you stay asleep. If you wake up and are too hot, stick your feet and hands out from under the covers. The body uses the extremities of your hands and feet as thermoregulatory mechanisms, and they offer us a quick way to heat up or cool down our core temperature. If you are experiencing hot flushes due to perimenopause or menopause, please see p. 198.

What this Looks Like for Me

Despite being a person who feels the cold easily, I don't have any heating in my bedroom, I sleep with the window open and wear loose cotton sleepwear. I will have a hot shower or bath if I am finding it harder to wind down for any reason, and this always helps.

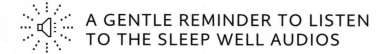

A GENTLE REMINDER TO LISTEN TO THE SLEEP WELL AUDIOS

You can access these audios for FREE with the passcode ISLEEPWELL on www.thepositivehabit.com.

Please remember to listen to the instructions for listening to guarantee maximum benefits.

MORNING MEDITATION

Please listen each morning to 'Start Your Day in Stillness – Intention-Setting Morning Meditation' to slow down your thoughts before the day commences.

AFTERNOON OR EVENING REST RITUAL

Please listen to 'Seven-Minute Rest Ritual' each afternoon and/or evening.

NIGHT-TIME HYPNOTHERAPY – WEEK FIVE: HABIT FIVE

This is the most important track to listen to. Each week there are new subconscious suggestions to help to reinforce the corresponding weekly habit and the following key insights.

To Get Back to Sleep if You Wake Up

You can listen to your night-time audio again, if necessary, but with time you will not need to do this. The Sleep Well Formula (Breathe + Imagine + Experience = Faith) which you are learning on a subconscious level every time you listen to your weekly audios will become automatic. Please also listen to the '4, 7, 8 Breathing' audio and train yourself to do this in the middle of the night should you awaken.

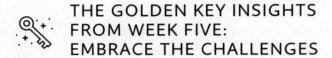

THE GOLDEN KEY INSIGHTS FROM WEEK FIVE: EMBRACE THE CHALLENGES

✦ Embracing your subjective sleep challenges now is worth the effort, and the reward is a sustainable shift in your relationship with sleep. You will enter into a lifelong love affair with sleep. It will see you through your toughest times, it will keep you healthy and wise and it will always bring out your brightest, lightest self.

✦ Whatever your sleep challenge is, continue to apply the **Sleep Well Formula (Breathe + Imagine + Experience = Faith)** and you will improve the effectiveness of your sleep. It won't be perfect, but it will most certainly be better.

✦ Remember the two-arrow parable. Many situations are out of your control, but your response is always within your grasp.

✦ If you believe you meet the criteria for insomnia please seek medical assistance. The criteria are on p. 191.

✦ Diurnal cortisol slopes refer to the release of cortisol over the course of 24 hours. A healthy release of cortisol spikes shortly after awakening and then slowly decreases as the day goes on with low levels at night, allowing for a smooth transition to sleep.

- ✦ Re-reading your sleep contract is a helpful thing to do at this stage as a way to keep your motivation levels high. It is normal to feel resistance arising when you are making even positive changes in your life. Be gentle with yourself.

- ✦ Habit Five is 'Optimise your light and temperature exposure'.

To maximise the benefits of this programme, I encourage you not to begin reading Week Six until you have listened to the 'Week Five: Habit Five' night-time audio for a minimum of seven nights in total.

Congratulations again on getting over the halfway mark. I am so proud of your progress. The image of your best-slept self is getting clearer and clearer each time you look in the mirror.

As always, acknowledge all progress and be compassionate to yourself on the days your sleep habits are less than perfect. The main thing is to keep going and do your best.

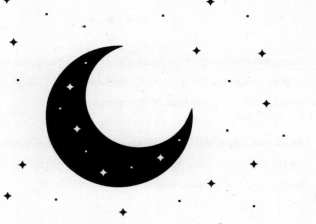

SLEEP STRENGTH ONE - PRESENCE

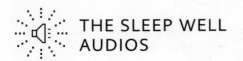

THE SLEEP WELL AUDIOS

All audios are available to download on www.thepositivehabit.com with the password ISLEEPWELL.

✦ **Tonight, please start listening to 'Week Six: Habit Six' of your Sleep Well audios. Please listen to this audio for a minimum of seven nights. Please do not skip ahead to Week Seven until you have listened for a full seven days.**

✦ **Please also continue to listen to your morning meditation and your rest ritual tracks each day.**

✦ ✦ ✦

Measure Your Sleep

BEFORE YOU BEGIN Week Six of the Sleep Well Programme, please take a moment to rate your sleep. On a scale of 0 to 10, how well have you slept in the last week? (0 is 'terribly' and 10 is 'very well'.) Please use the image on the opposite page to mark where you feel you are on this scale.

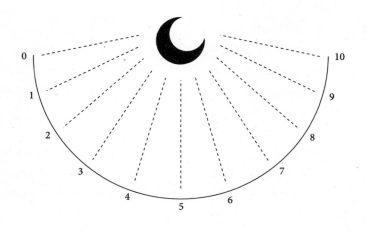

✦ ✦ ✦

A Poem to Fall Asleep With

The Oak

Live thy Life,
Young and old,
Like yon oak,
Bright in spring,
Living gold;

Summer-rich
Then; and then
Autumn-changed
Soberer-hued
Gold again.

All his leaves
Fall'n at length,
Look, he stands,
Trunk and bough
Naked strength.

ALFRED, LORD TENNYSON

A Story to Fall Asleep With

ONE DAY LAST summer, in the stunning and scorched Tuscan hills, I was frustrated. I had been feeling anxious for a number of days and it seemed to be for no tangible reason. I was in a beautiful and idyllic landscape surrounded by my loving family. I had no cause to feel uneasy, and yet this ambiguous anxiety lingered. I felt stagnant, like the heat of the sun. I was irritated at not being present enough to enjoy my well-earned holiday. Anxiety can raise its head when you least expect it; recrimination and resistance will only fuel it.

The intense Tuscan heat had been causing me to wake up at 5 a.m. for over a week. I naively thought this would be a positive. I'd have more time for meditation, yoga and exercise before it became too hot. However, I was going to bed just before midnight, leaving me with a meagre five hours of sleep. I was totally exhausted by midday and was no fun at all for the rest of the day.

The cause of my fearful state was clearly not coming from my surroundings, which were lush and serene. Nor was there a psychological component. It was the lack of sleep that had me so edgy. Retrospect lends clarity to situations that are so obvious in hindsight. Yet when you are going through them, they can remain a total mystery. Especially when it comes to sleep deprivation. My brain was so depleted and clouded my vision of something that was so obvious.

One day, I recall sunbathing in my disquiet when I stumbled upon an Eckhart Tolle video on YouTube. It was called 'The Importance of Conscious Breathing' and rather reluctantly I hit Play even though I egotistically thought to myself, *I already know all this* ... However, as I listened and took a conscious breath, I was transformed in an instant. My anxiety melted along with everything else, and I was back home in the eternal now.

The words Tolle spoke that elevated me so swiftly were 'Just to remind you, as I am sure everybody knows [my ego was satisfied!], a quick way of dropping out of thought is to take one conscious breath.' Startlingly simple. Nothing new, yet they were the exact words that I needed to hear at that precise moment.

I woke up that day, despite my exhaustion, and I was able to truly enjoy the countryside around me. I saw the patchwork of olive groves, vineyards and tall poplar trees as if for the first time. That night, I slept well. The next morning, I woke very refreshed, having had a lie-in until 7.30 a.m. As a lion, it was important to let my inner bear out.

Welcome to Week Six

SO FAR IN the Sleep Well Programme, you have made a decision to sleep well, explored your sleep story, examined your waking and sleeping self from a personal and scientific perspective and embraced your challenges. You are pretty amazing and deserve to sleep well and live fully. The next three weeks of the programme take a slightly different approach. We are moving our focus from the process of getting to sleep and staying asleep and into three strengths that will uplift your life and deepen your sleep.

The three strengths that you have already been subliminally learning about each night are presence, patience and peace. Who does not want more of these in their lives? At the end of each week, I will provide you with reflective journaling exercises to deepen your understanding of these strengths and also positive affirmations that will reinforce them in a practical way.

The Three Core Sleep Strengths

THE CORE SLEEP strengths naturally create a feeling of harmony within yourself and with the world. Consider these strengths as a calming blanket at night and an empowering, motivating energy during the day.

✦ Presence: how to live in the eternal now

✦ Patience: how to practise kindness and compassion

✦ Peace: how to feel content with who you are

Within each of these strengths, you will find a subset of skills that support them, as outlined above.

In positive psychology, 'positive affect' is known as the experience of a range of positive emotions, such as happiness, joy, love and gratitude. The culmination of regularly feeling these emotional states has been shown to reduce early death by nearly 20 per cent.[65]

You don't have to be a neuroscientist to know that positive emotions feel good. The problem is that positive emotions flow through your system quickly, unlike negative emotions that hijack your nervous system. Happier emotions are often more subtle and in a busy mind they can go unnoticed.

You need to soak in well-being to maximise your positive affect and increase your longevity.

The three core sleep strengths that you are building as you sleep, via your hypnotherapy audios, will help you to do just that. A pilot study conducted in the Department of Psychology and Neuroscience at the University of Texas on hypnotic relaxation therapy to increase well-being measured the participants' levels of positive emotions and symptoms of anxiety and distress before and after the study.[66] The results showed that as many as 71 per cent of participants improved their levels of overall positive affect after only a five-week intervention. Being able to use self-hypnosis audios and relaxation techniques at home added to the overall success of the programme.

Dr David Spiegel from Stanford University has dedicated much of his 40-year career to highlighting the benefits of hypnosis on many issues including sleep. In an interview with his colleague and host of the *Huberman Lab Podcast*, Andrew Huberman, he said, 'Hypnosis can be very helpful for dissociating somatic reactions from psychological reactions and in controlling the mind-body in relation to stress. It's very helpful for people to get to sleep. I'm getting emails from people who have said, "I haven't slept right in fifteen years, and now for the first time, I can sleep at night."'[67]

It is also worth reminding you again that the night-time hypnotherapy audios are helping you on a subliminal level. As your sleep improves, you don't need to consciously work everything out; your deep sleep and dreams are working away in the background for you.

The first core sleep strength of presence echoes and reinforces our work up to now, in particular Week Three: Your Waking Self. We will begin now, the only moment you have, and explore the first strength in more detail. It is important that you work consecutively through the strengths in the order they are delivered: each builds on the previous one.

Presence

'THE NAKED STRENGTH' referred to in Tennyson's poem at the start of this chapter is, to my mind, presence. This strength is one you can't see or touch, and yet its power can be felt everywhere. Presence emerges from letting go of attachment to the conditioned mind.

**Presence is the energy you bring to the world
when you are awake and have slept soundly.**

In this section, I ask you to examine your relationship with the present moment and how you can improve this relationship both during the day and when you drift to sleep at night. You will learn how deep your breath is and how one conscious breath can transform your emotional state in an instant. To be present is to know that you are alive and to know who you are. It is the quality of stillness that you bring to all your actions. It is the quality of loving reality as it is and people as they are, including yourself. It is freedom. It is joy. It is always here. It is now.

How do you allow this state of consciousness to induce golden slumber? Presence.

Presence is also the fundamental energy you need to wake up.

PSYCHOLOGICAL TIME

To help you with this idea of creating presence for both sleep and wakefulness, Eckhart Tolle divides time into two separate concepts. The first is 'psychological time'. This is when your mind is not present but is consumed with thoughts of the past or the future or caught up in a current life situation, for example fretting over a work issue. You have drifted from the eternal now, which is a sense of timelessness and a focus on the immediate experience of the present moment. Psychological time, by its very nature, creates anxiety and pulls you from presence. Through a lack of awareness, you begin to believe that psychological time is your life.

Generally speaking, if you are caught up in the past, you are more likely to experience regret and rumination. You could be yearning for a time in your life when you perceived yourself to be happier – for example when your children were small, or you first fell in love. Obsessive thoughts of the future could be a false perception that some moment yet to come will be brighter than this moment. That moment never arises, and yet you cling to the idea that you will be happy when ... you live in the sun, meet a new partner, have a child or reach spiritual enlightenment. A compulsive need to over-plan is often an attempt to control the uncertainty of life, which is, of course, futile.

Making friends with uncertainty allows you to accept the present moment as it is.

This is not to say that you let go of organising and planning. This is of course necessary to function. You can plan for the future while still retaining presence. You are aware you are in planning mode, and you can come back out of it when the job is done. This is useful both lying in bed and during the day.

Psychological time can also create an over-identification of the roles you play and the responsibilities they bring. For example, if you lose your job, you also lose your sense of self – without a title you don't know who you are.

CLOCK TIME

'Clock time', Tolle's second concept of time, is highly practical, and it will liberate your mind from racing thoughts, whether you are drifting to sleep or in the midst of your working day.

Clock time simply means an awareness of the moment and where you need to be or what you need to be doing. Sometimes this doing is nothing and simply 'being', and you can allow time to flow uninterrupted. For example, if you are walking in the woods and you don't have to be somewhere afterwards, there is no rush, and you can literally take your time. However, if you have a flight to catch later that day, you will evidently need to plan to leave at the appropriate time to make sure you are not rushed.

To operate in the world of work, to have friends, and to be a reliable human being, clock time is essential.

Personally, I'm very organised. I thrive on utilising time effectively, and clock time, rather than confining me, permits me to be present. For example, when I run a wellness retreat, the timetable is very structured (including periods to rest and reflect) and this framework ensures that I maximise the time I have to help my group. The structure liberates us all to bring our full selves to the moment without concerns about what is happening later or having 'enough time'. Time expands rather than shrinks. A week's retreat feels like a mini-lifetime, a world all of its own.

A question to ask yourself regularly, and especially when going to sleep, if you notice your mind racing is: 'Am I now in psychological time or clock time?'

When you are lying in bed, what do you have to do? Nothing. Where do you have to be? Nowhere. Now is a moment of non-action and letting go. Your only purpose is to rest and relax. Bliss.

Asking yourself the above question often is a direct path to presence. It is a highly effective way of not over-identifying with external events in your life that have the potential to create drama. Many years ago, in my early twenties, I used to watch depressing soap operas. Each one was grimmer than the last. I compulsively watched the characters struggle from one personal disaster to another and I witnessed them create much of their own downfall (although I didn't see it like that then) by reacting and contributing to the endless stress in their lives. One day, I just stopped watching. I liberated myself. Living in 'clock time' means you turn the drama off in your own life.

Will the stress still be there? Yes. The difference is that you are no longer amplifying the inevitable challenges of being alive. From those daily minor irritants to a more major traumatic event in your life, you are able to witness the stress and to feel the emotions without getting lost in them. Reframing stress into a healthy opportunity for positive growth builds emotional resilience, and how you perceive stress changes how it manifests physically.

From the frustrating to heartbreaking events in your life, you give them space to unfold. Yet they are not pervasive or all-consuming. You take a literal and metaphorical step back. This step is not representative of denial but a much-needed space to allow a solution to emerge. For example, you still have the capacity to enjoy meeting a friend without being consumed by your problems. Clock time gives an immediate sense of perspective. It teaches you to do one thing at a time.

Be extremely patient with this concept. In a world of multitasking, it needs consistent practice. An example of this is a client of mine, let's call her Andrea, who was very worried about her daughter who had been bullied at school. The situation was clearly distressing, but her daughter was now in a new school and settling in well.

I had taught Andrea the principle of clock vs psychological time in one of our sessions. The next time I saw Andrea she told me that she was out for a walk in her favourite place in nature and found herself completely lost in worrying about her daughter. She had visions of her being isolated for the rest of her life (psychological time), she was catastrophising and very stressed. However, she caught herself just in time and was aware that, ironically, she was *not aware* of her surroundings (clock time). She said to herself, 'Look at the flowers,' and felt an immediate sense of ease. Coming home to presence meant she was able to reassure herself that staying calm and positive was the best way to help her daughter to regain her confidence and flourish in the world. When you do this, please notice just how empowering it is.

INNER AND OUTER WORLDS

In addition to having two time frames, you also inhabit two worlds. The first is your external world. This is one of form and it is what is generally referred to as 'life'. The external world is the roles you have and the responsibilities of family and work. The second world you inhabit is your internal one, and this is a sacred space that is found in stillness.

> **In order to sleep peacefully, connect to yourself through stillness each day.**

This connection is created through non-doing and rest. Meditation, hypnotherapy, yoga, chi gong and other ancient spiritual practices that encourage us to unify the mind and body are all wonderful access points to stillness. The internal world of presence is a terrain rarely visited; however, this is shifting, and it is estimated that globally between two hundred and five hundred million people meditate.[68] The morning meditation and rest ritual included in this programme are designed to help you come home to this inner space often. Taking a few minutes to surrender to stillness before and during a busy day will unite your body and mind. You are training yourself to be at peace in your waking day so you can make a smooth transition into sleep when the time comes.

If you do not consciously take time to connect to your internal world, then it is likely that any fears and negative thoughts you had during the day (but were too distracted to notice) will rise up as soon as you close your eyes. If you do drift off quickly you are likely to be jolted wide awake later in the night or in those early hours of the morning, when it is too early to rise. The thoughts, fears, anxieties, hopes and dreams all come tumbling in, a tidal wave of tension. These anxieties have at last got your attention, like a child who has been desperately trying to speak to you all day. This is the time when your thoughts need to slow down, not speed up.

When it comes to sleep, your thoughts matter. Every thought has a corresponding neurochemical response in your body. A stressful thought will spike cortisol and adrenaline, which activates your rather inaptly named 'sympathetic' nervous system. This is the body's stress response, and it will of course make going to sleep and staying asleep difficult. Your brain perceives stressful thoughts as genuine and immediate threats, and it will give you a shot of adrenaline to help you fight or flee this potential aggressor. You are lying in bed, you do not want to fight anyone or run anywhere, but the trouble is your brain does not know this.

Work-related stress is particularly likely to send your nervous system into a spiral. The reason many people lose sleep over work is that it is directly linked to our survival – most of us depend on our income to live, and if we feel we are not performing at work, this will have a direct impact on feeling secure. Your breathing and heart rate increase. Your frustration and fear are now stronger, and falling asleep is definitely not a priority in the primitive part of your brain. It is designed for survival and this perceived stress is a threat. Why would it go to sleep?

POSITIVE IMAGINATION

On the other hand, soothing, happy thoughts release serotonin and oxytocin to activate the parasympathetic system, also known as the rest and digest system. As you are already aware, the Sleep Well Formula (Breathe + Imagine + Experience = Faith) is helping you to do this each night.

For now, try this thought experiment with me. Think of a positive memory in your life. Perhaps it was when you graduated from college, a celebration such as a wedding or a big birthday, the first time you fell in love or, if you have children, the birth of your baby.

When you have selected a happy moment in your life, allow all of your senses to catapult you back to that scene. Pay attention to the details. The people in the room, the sounds, the colours, the aromas. Reach out and touch something. Can you recall what you or other people were wearing?

This culmination of thoughts creates a positive memory and if you really allow that memory to soak in this will have a neurochemical response in the body, releasing both serotonin and dopamine.

I am recalling the first time I looked into the eyes of my son. I remember his little eyes and the light that shone from him. I knew there were other people in the room, but I only saw him. The longer I stay with this image, the more I produce life-enhancing neurochemicals that will help me to sleep.

Research shows us that the release of positive neurochemicals is conducive to activating the sleep hormone gamma-aminobutyric acid (GABA).[69] GABA is an inhibitory neurotransmitter and plays a pivotal role in reducing neural activity and creating relaxation.[70]

It acts as a buffer between being over-stimulated and sleep, so the more GABA you have, the sooner you get to sleep. It has been shown that GABA also promotes slow-wave, deep sleep.

Deep sleep is the dishwasher of the brain, flushing away toxins, replenishing energy, helping store memories, regulating emotions, boosting the immune system and balancing hormones.

The interplay between these 'happy hormones' GABA and melatonin (a critical hormone in regulating the sleep–wake cycle) all helps to open the door to a regenerative night's sleep. The more relaxed and content you feel before bed, the better. Habit Two, 'Create a "blissful hour" 60-minute bedtime routine', in your Sleep Well Programme will create the necessary level of GABA to ensure your brain is getting the deep clean it needs.

The Sleep Well Programme is training you to become your own pharmacist, dispensing the exact neurochemicals that you need to induce rest and relaxation (serotonin) and above all what you need to induce a beautiful night's sleep (melatonin). No prescription is necessary.

Can you recall the How Present Are You questionnaire you answered in Week One: Your Decision to Sleep Well? Please go back to p. 33 now and notice whether your answers have shifted.

PRESENCE AND SLEEP ARE INNATE

The strength of presence is within you already. Witness a baby and observe how they engage with the world with awe and wonder.

When they feel relaxed and safe, a baby can gaze at a tree or a flower for hours. As John O'Donohue said, 'experience each day as a sacred gift woven around the heart of wonder.' A baby personifies presence, and you were once that baby.

> **As you sleep well, it is this deeper part of you that is reawakening.**

There is no need to doubt or cling to presence – it is here. It is the energy in your body that continues to move when you are motionless. Close your eyes for a moment and focus on bringing complete stillness to your body, wait until the mind settles and you will feel this inner energy. It's subtle, but there is an energy that is always alive within you. In your waking state or sleep, your breath is always flowing consistently, bringing you home. However, when your mind is infected with too many thoughts, like a virus, you become compromised, and you lose sight of who you are and what truly matters. You can become obsessed with insignificant details and suffer from repetitive thoughts that activate the stress response. A mind that is crammed with thoughts is like a fire that rages. It sucks all the oxygen out of the atmosphere. Being burnt out is having nothing left to give.

Your breath is your pathway to presence, to your home. You need to keep coming back time and time again, day after day and night after night. The reason that one conscious breath was so wonderfully effective on that hot day in Italy was not a coincidence. I was able to return to presence ONLY because of the years of mindfulness, breath work, meditation, hypnotherapy and yoga practice that I had already spent on this one concept – uniting my body and mind and being in the one place at the one time. This is why I could switch from Tolle's psychological time (worrying about the future, ruminating on the past, feeling anxious) into clock time (presence, the eternal now) so smoothly. The more you practise, the shorter the gaps between distraction and presence and between wakefulness and sleep.

THE STORIES WE TELL OURSELVES

Living in presence illuminates the truth of who you are: pure consciousness. When you are present, your personal history, coupled with your ego, fades into the background and you come home to who you are. You are not the story of your past or the projection of your future. You are energy that exists only here and now. You are never more true to the essence of your being than when you still your mind.

To still the mind takes practice, and as we discussed in Week Three, this can be done both formally through meditation and informally with mindfulness. Either way, the deeper level of who you are is always at peace and the surface level is often seeking acknowledgement or drama. You know you have left presence when you become consumed with thought. One thought leads to another, and before you know it, you have created a narrative. As you learnt in Week Two: Your Sleep Story, paying attention to these stories that you play on repeat in your mind is essential. Often the story is stale and arises from hurt or injustice in the past. Often you may not even be aware of this thought pattern and how much it shapes your life. I have seen many of these patterns in my clinic over the years.

The most common ones are:

✦ 'I am always the one in my family who has to do everything.'

- ✦ 'I work so hard, and I am never acknowledged fully.'

- ✦ 'I give so much and other people take me for granted.'

- ✦ 'I am never going to have the confidence or energy to pursue my dream.'

- ✦ 'I have never known what my purpose in life is.'

Becoming still is reclaiming your own consciousness. You begin to see the story for what it is: a fabrication of the mind. You say to your thoughts, *Move over, make some space – for me to be.* Consider your mind like a beautiful house that is crammed with boxes, and these boxes are crammed with old belongings you no longer use. In fact, you are not even sure what is in most of them. The multitude of boxes hides both the magnificence and the potential that your house has to offer. When people come to visit, despite the expanse of the home, there is nowhere for them to sit. The overthinking mind is this clutter, and by engaging with this programme, you are doing a much-needed clear-out.

DEEP BREATHING

Slowing down your breath by practising deep diaphragmatic breathing, also known as belly breathing, changes your life. Try this now.

- ✦ Set a timer for one minute.

- ✦ Without changing your breath, count how many normal breaths you take in 60 seconds.

The average number is anywhere between 12 and 16.[71] Dr Sat Bir Singh Khalsa (his story is in Week Three) is an associate professor of medicine at Harvard Medical School, and a pioneer in the research of yoga. He states the optimum number of breaths per minute is between four and six. There is a growing mountain of data to support what the ancient mystics knew thousands of years ago: slow breathing promotes better emotional and physical health.[72]

Yogic breathing, also known as pranayama, is the ancient art of controlled slow and deep diaphragmatic breaths. It is often performed in conjunction with meditation and the physical component of yoga for its spiritual and health-enhancing effects. The benefits include higher heart rate variability, improved autonomic function and increased emotional regulation. Simply put, the slower you breathe, the calmer you feel, the less reactive you are and the stronger and more able your immune system is to fight infection and disease.[73]

Marketing images for yoga often portray super slim, fully flexible, beautifully toned and tanned people in postures that remain impossible for most of us. Yet yoga is for everyone who wants to unite their body and mind, to be both emotionally and physically strong. Yoga is not an activity, it is a philosophy, a lifestyle. The movement combined with the breath work offers a holistic and preventative approach to many of the lifestyle and non-communicable diseases that are the number one cause of death today.[74] I hope you have had an opportunity to introduce some gentle yoga into your life since Week Four (if you don't already have a practice). Remember, the bridge pose is a great one to do as part of Habit Two (the 'blissful hour' bedtime routine).

Deeper and slower breaths will become your standard mode of operating and not something you desperately pull out at the last moment before you speak in public, get on a plane or have an awkward conversation with your boss. In these moments, without prior practice, it is often too late, and the body is already in a state of acute stress.

The hypnotherapy audios coupled with the yogic resting ritual included in this programme are training you to change how you breathe. Your deeper and slower breathing will help you to cope with life's inevitable challenges and to sleep peacefully at night from a stance of loving presence.

Please continue to slow and deepen your breathing and then time your breaths again at the end of this programme. You will, I am sure, notice a difference.

One Conscious Breath
As you slow your breath, you will inevitably experience a higher level of consciousness. When you are truly present, a wonderful sense of comfort, safety and happiness arises. One conscious breath is all it takes to reconnect your mind to your body. One conscious breath is all you need to focus on as you let go of everything else not contained in this precious moment – the only one you have. Your stress and anxiety can melt away and you can sleep peacefully, no matter what challenges you face.

Try this simple experiment for me now:

✦ Allow yourself to dwell on a concern or issue you may have, something small or significant.

+ Take one full and deep conscious belly breath. Place all your attention on the inhale and the exhale, feel the breath as it reaches your lungs and observe it as you exhale.

+ Right here and now that stressor does not exist; it is simply a thought in your mind.

+ If you can intervene before another thought starts and creates an avalanche, you are free. Your 'house' is becoming clear again.

As we learnt in Week Three there are benefits from mind wandering, such as increased creativity and solutions to problems arising when you least expect them. Still, disconnecting your thoughts from the moment, where you are and what you are doing on a consistent basis comes at an emotional cost. A seminal Harvard study conducted in 2010 by researchers and psychologists Killingsworth and Gilbert uncovered that 46.9 per cent of the time, our minds have wandered away from presence.[75]

For almost half of our lives, we are asleep to reality.

The study used a special 'track your happiness' app to gather data by randomly asking the participants where they were and if their mind was connected to what they were doing. They found that people were most present when making love, exercising or engaging in conversation. I remain unclear as to how the participants responded when they were making love! They were least connected to the now when resting, working or using a computer.

The study went on to show that as little as 4.6 per cent of our happiness is actually connected to the activity we are doing – but this figure is much higher if we are present while doing it. The lead researchers said, 'How often our minds leave the present and where they go is a greater predictor of our happiness than the activities in which we are engaged.' Presence allows you to be equally happy when you are at home doing the dishes and when you are dining out in an exquisite restaurant. Your breath is the bridge between mind and body: it is always here, always present.

PRESENCE IN RELATIONSHIPS

Do you spend enough time with the people in your life who matter most? Depending on what life stage you are at and the level of your responsibilities, you may simply not have the time you would like to prioritise these relationships. The research is clear that isolation and loneliness are seriously damaging to your health, and a lack of connection shortens your life.[76]

As you fall in love with sleep, you will find that your energy increases, and as your energy increases, you have more to spend with the people you love. It is wise to look at the relationships you have in your life, all the way from your casual acquaintances to your closest connections, and ask the following questions:

✦ How do I feel in the presence of this person?

✦ Do I feel that I bring out the best in myself when I am in their company?

✦ Do I feel belittled or smaller?

✦ How do I think people feel when they leave my company?

Are there members of your family you would like to have a better relationship with but find it hard? The feeling of being disconnected from loved ones is what keeps many people awake at night. Family tensions can run deep, and it takes immense presence and courage to ameliorate them. Rest assured, the more you work on loving the challenging parts of yourself, the more you will be able to share this with family members you may find difficult.

Most of our conflicts and confrontations and lack of empathy come from an unresolved internal conflict. The most important relationship you have in your life is the one with yourself. Eckhart Tolle often points out that if you believe you are enlightened, you should spend time with your family of origin and notice how easily you can be triggered. He says, 'Human interaction can be hell. Or it can be a great spiritual practice.' If you find yourself feeling irritated, angry or disappointed with a loved one, can you use this energy to deepen the relationship rather than potentially destroy it? The energy of staying present to the difficult emotions in yourself will help them to soften.

The relationships in your life, especially that with your partner, if you have one, provide the richest soil to learn about your idiosyncrasies. Many of us make the mistake of trying to change the people we love to match our version of the world. We think, 'If only they were more patient/affectionate/fun/successful/confident' or 'Maybe if they were less needy/aggressive/moody/difficult/boring, then the relationship would be better.' In reference to Jungian psychology, the shadow self is an element of your character that you have repressed or shut down due to what emotional support – or indeed lack of support – you had as a child and adolescent. It is often the qualities in others that we find most intolerable that are the very things that we have suppressed in ourselves.

Self-knowledge leads to accountability, and it allows you to be present with the people you love. You are aware of why you feel the emotions you do, and as a result you are not controlled by them.

Self-liberation allows you to set free the people you love.

Trying to change another person is a form of control that often stems from a fear of being abandoned. This lack of presence is very damaging to the relationship, because the underlying message is 'I cannot love you as you are. My love is conditional.'

When you give from a place that is already full, love is abundant, you have enough, and it keeps on renewing itself. You love a person for who they are and not the fairytale version of them that you have created in your head. You do not require that you get that love back at a time or in a fashion that you dictate. You have the presence to observe how their love is returned in subtle ways, for example the full tank of petrol in the car, the tiptoeing through the hall so as not to wake you, the refusal to say, 'I told you so' when you make a mistake. It is in silence that love is expressed most loudly.

Dr Rick Hanson said, 'If we move through our day with an open awareness of the good things around us, we correct the brain's built-in negativity bias.' Choose to see the best in everyone that you meet, bring your attention to their good qualities, and they will shine. The 'Pygmalion effect' is a psychological phenomenon based on the Greek myth of Pygmalion, a sculptor who fell so deeply in love with a statue he created that it came to life. When you see the best in a person, they start to see it too.

This is particularly important when it comes to children and adolescents who look to you to guide them to make sense of themselves and the world. For example, if a parent worries that her child lacks confidence, the child will pick up on this projection and feel a sense of inadequacy. The situation becomes amplified, not better. The unspoken negative thoughts infect the child with self-doubt. Presence allows you to transform worry into compassion: love in action.

The depth of your sleeping, your breath and your presence all happen simultaneously. When you live in the eternal now, you are that person who makes others feel that they are the only person in the world. Your attention is focused on who is right in front of you and you hold space for people without judgement. As you listen, you have no agenda and people are consistently drawn to you. Opportunities you never dreamt of (or perhaps you did) start to manifest. Your best-slept self lives in your presence. As your consciousness shifts to a higher level you become part of a unique movement of enlightened beings. You are waking up to who you truly are – presence.

From this place, you are ready to explore the second sleep strength, which is one most of us, including myself, need more of – patience.

✦ ✦ ✦

Reflective Journaling Prompts

✦ Recall a period in your life when you were predominantly living in the moment. This could be as a child or later as a young adult. A time when you felt truly alive and connected to the now. Write about it in as much detail as possible.

✦ When during your regular routine are you most present?

✦ How committed are you to changing how you breathe? Do you believe it will help you to sleep more peacefully and live more in the present moment?

✦ ✦ ✦

Affirmations to Repeat

✦ 'I am here. I am now. I am presence.'

✦ 'I am the eternal now.'

✦ 'I look for the good in everyone I encounter.'

✦ ✦ ✦

Build Your Sleep Well Habits

CONTINUE WITH THE habits you've formed in the previous weeks:

✦ Habit One: You go to sleep and wake up at roughly the same time every day.

✦ Habit Two: You have a 'blissful hour' bedtime routine.

✦ Habit Three: You move your body.

✦ Habit Four: You reduce your alcohol and caffeine intake.

✦ Habit Five: You optimise your light and temperature exposure.

Keep building as you go, and remember, a lot of the Sleep Well habits only require small tweaks to your life for significant rewards.

HABIT SIX

Eat Mindfully and at Regular Times

BRINGING PRESENCE TO eating is essentially what is known as mindful eating. This ensures that, just like your breath, you slow down your eating, you savour the food and you embody a sense of appreciation for the food you have. You will eat less and enjoy your food more.

My dog Rosie, needless to say, has no sleep issues, but she is permanently hungry and not so mindful when she eats! She knows the times of her feeding schedule without ever having to look at a clock. Five to ten minutes before she is due to be fed, Rosie will start to tell me it is her breakfast or dinner time. Her body has been trained to expect food at that time each day, and believe me, it is not a good idea to keep her waiting!

Your body is no different. It responds well to being fed at the same times each day. However, when you are disconnected from your body, you will miss those signals. If you are caught up in a work deadline or personal situation, you leave yourself hungry and can end up overeating later in the day, which leads to disrupted sleep.

The human growth hormone (HGH) that is responsible for cell regeneration and how our bodies collect fat (especially around the stomach area) is released in a large bolus in the first half of the night. Going to bed at the same time means that you don't miss out on this early sleep and hence are also helping yourself to maintain a healthy weight. In the same way that light exposure has an impact on your circadian rhythm, so too does the time you eat. When you eat erratically you interfere with the sleep–wake cycle. Eating at inappropriate times, such as late at night, is incredibly disruptive to the quality of your sleep, as it puts pressure on your digestive system when it needs to prioritise rest.

Quality sleep is essential to regulate the hormones ghrelin and leptin, which control your appetite. Ghrelin is the hormone that stimulates hunger and leptin is the highly important hormone that sends messages of satiety to the brain. If you are sleep deprived, you are more likely to crave high-calorie foods to help combat fatigue. You also miss the message from gut to brain that you are full.

If your sleep is poor, your appetite will increase, and you will find it harder to lose weight. It makes sense that when your energy is depleted you turn to food and caffeine to try and boost it. The following three practices will help you to make healthy food choices that support your great night's sleep.

+ Avoid eating for three hours before going to sleep. Sleeping on a full stomach will put pressure on your digestive system and your insulin resistance increases at night. Snacking in front of the TV ensures those extra calories are stored as fat that you don't burn off.

+ Stick to eating at the same time each day. Regular eating times support the master clock's signals to your sleep–wake cycle. Your body thrives on routine and your digestive system will find its rhythm each day as it has an expectation of when it will be fed.

+ Eat foods high in magnesium, melatonin and calcium to aid sleep. Some examples of these are:

  ◇ Almonds: melatonin and magnesium

  ◇ Warm milk: calcium, vitamin D, melatonin and tryptophan – the serotonin produced by tryptophan is converted into more melatonin. By increasing the levels of melatonin in your body, tryptophan promotes relaxation and calmness, making it easier to fall asleep and stay asleep. Childhood associations can also help induce a feeling of comfort.

- ◇ Walnuts: melatonin, serotonin and magnesium.

- ◇ Other foods rich in magnesium are spinach, black beans, avocado, salmon, dark chocolate, pumpkin seeds, and quinoa. Include these in your dinner to promote good sleep naturally.

- ◇ Foods rich in calcium: dairy products (milk, cheese, yoghurt), leafy greens (kale, spinach, cabbage), tofu, sardines, soybeans, sesame seeds and figs.

- ◇ Foods rich in melatonin: turkey, chicken, tuna, eggs, lentils, oats, pumpkin seeds, sesame seeds and sunflower seeds.

✦ Portion size is also important. A light breakfast will give you the energy you need to be alert and to help you wake up. You don't want to have too full a stomach early in the day, as your energy will be diverted to digesting food and this can cause you to feel lethargic. Leave your largest meal and most of your carbohydrates until your final meal of the day, as this will help to induce a feeling of drowsiness and comfort, which are both conducive to making sleep effortless.

Over time your eating patterns create predictable autonomic timing that causes wakefulness when you need to be alert and sleepiness when it is time to sleep.

What this Looks Like for Me
I eat mainly a plant-based Mediterranean diet, rich in colour and variety. I eat a lot of the foods mentioned above, such as almonds, seeds, eggs and yoghurt. I eat breakfast about 60–90 minutes

after rising and also have my first intake of caffeine then. I eat lunch and dinner at roughly the same time every day; this will vary depending on the season. In summer, I eat and go to bed later. I aim to leave a fasting window of 14 hours between my last meal and my breakfast. I have to consistently remind myself to slow down when I am eating and to bring presence with me to the table.

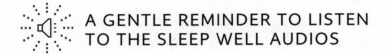

A GENTLE REMINDER TO LISTEN TO THE SLEEP WELL AUDIOS

You can access these audios for FREE with the passcode ISLEEPWELL on www.thepositivehabit.com.

Please remember to listen to the instructions for listening to guarantee maximum benefits.

MORNING MEDITATION

Please listen each morning to 'Start Your Day in Stillness – Intention-Setting Morning Meditation' to slow down your thoughts, before the day commences.

AFTERNOON OR EVENING REST RITUAL

Please listen to 'Seven-Minute Rest Ritual' each afternoon and/or evening.

NIGHT-TIME HYPNOTHERAPY – WEEK SIX: HABIT SIX

This is the most important track to listen to. Each week there are new subconscious suggestions to help to reinforce the corresponding weekly habit and the following key insights.

To Get Back to Sleep if You Wake Up

You can listen to your night-time audio again, if necessary, but with time you will not need to do this. The Sleep Well Formula (Breathe + Imagine + Experience = Faith) which you are learning on a subconscious level every time you listen to your weekly audios will become automatic. Please also listen to the '4, 7, 8 Breathing' audio and train yourself to do this in the middle of the night should you awaken.

THE GOLDEN KEY INSIGHTS FROM WEEK SIX: SLEEP STRENGTH ONE – PRESENCE

✦ Presence is the energy you bring to the world when you are awake and have slept soundly.

✦ Eckhart Tolle's psychological time is when your mind is not present but is consumed with thoughts of the past or the future or caught up in a current life situation, for example worrying over a health concern, or your sleep!

✦ Clock time simply means an awareness of the moment and where you need to be or what you need to be doing. Sometimes this doing is nothing and simply 'being', and you can allow time to flow uninterrupted. You want to be in clock time when you are in bed – you are in bed.

✦ Focusing your imagination on happy thoughts releases serotonin and oxytocin to activate the parasympathetic system, also known as the rest and digest system. This is the perfect place for sleep to come to you.

- ✦ Slowing down your breath by practising deep diaphragmatic breathing, also known as belly breathing, changes your life. One conscious breath can be enough to cut through psychological time (worry) into clock time (presence).

- ✦ Please make sure to take the time to do your reflective journaling and repeat your presence affirmations.

- ✦ Your Habit this week is Habit Six – 'Eat mindfully and at regular times'.

To maximise the benefits of this programme, I encourage you not to begin reading Week Seven until you have listened to the 'Week Six– Habit Six' night-time audio for a minimum of seven nights in total.

I truly hope you have enjoyed learning about your sleep (and life) strength presence. Like Andrea, my client, be patient with yourself and fully acknowledge any 'aha' moments when you make the shift from the fog of thinking into the clarity of a still mind.

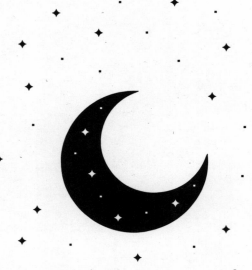

SLEEP STRENGTH TWO - PATIENCE

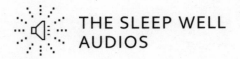

THE SLEEP WELL
AUDIOS

All audios are available to download on www.thepositivehabit.com with the password ISLEEPWELL.

✦ Tonight, please start listening to 'Week Seven: Habit Seven' of the Sleep Well audios. Please listen to this audio for a minimum of seven nights. Please do not skip ahead to Week Eight until you have listened for a full seven days.

✦ Please also continue to listen to your morning meditation and your rest ritual tracks each day.

✦ ✦ ✦

Measure Your Sleep

BEFORE YOU BEGIN Week Seven of the Sleep Well Programme, please take a moment to rate your sleep. On a scale of 0 to 10, how well have you slept in the last week? (0 is 'terribly' and 10 is 'very well'.) Please use the image on the opposite page to mark where you feel you are on this scale.

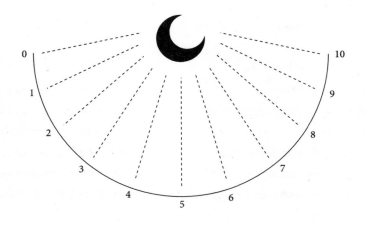

✦ ✦ ✦

A Poem to Fall Asleep With

Patience Taught by Nature

'O Dreary life!' we cry, 'O dreary life!'
And still, the generations of the birds
Sing through our sighing, and the flocks and herds
Serenely live while we are keeping strife
With Heaven's true purpose in us, as a knife
Against which we may struggle. Ocean girds
Unslackened the dry land: savannah-swards
Unweary sweep: hills watch, unworn; and rife
Meek leaves drop yearly from the forest trees,
To show, above, the unwasted stars that pass
In their old glory. O thou God of old!
Grant me some smaller grace than comes to these;—
But so much patience, as a blade of grass
Grows by contented through the heat and cold.

ELIZABETH BARRETT BROWNING 1806–1861

A Story to Fall Asleep With

THE TRUE STORY written below by Kent Nerburn, author of *Make Me an Instrument of Your Peace: Living in the Spirit of the Prayer of Saint Francis,* is a wonderful illustration of patience in practice. Kent is an American author who focuses on Native American spirituality. I am grateful to him for his permission to publish his story here.

✦ ✦ ✦

There was a time in my life twenty years ago when I was driving a cab for a living. It was a cowboy's life, a gambler's life, a life for someone who wanted no boss, constant movement and the thrill of a dice roll every time a new passenger got into the cab. What I didn't count on when I took the job was that it was also a ministry.

Because I drove the night shift, my cab became a rolling confessional. Passengers would climb in, sit behind me in total anonymity and tell me of their lives. We were like strangers on a train, the passengers and I, hurtling through the night, revealing intimacies we would never have dreamed of sharing during the brighter light of day. I encountered people whose lives amazed me, ennobled me, made me laugh and made me weep. And none of those lives touched me more than that of a woman I picked up late on a warm August night.

I was responding to a call from a small brick fourplex in a quiet part of town. I assumed I was being sent to pick up some partiers, or someone who had just had a fight with a lover, or someone going off to an early shift at some factory in the industrial part of town.

When I arrived at the address, the building was dark except for a single light in a ground-floor window. Under these circumstances, many drivers would just honk once or twice, wait a short minute, and then drive away. Too many bad possibilities awaited a driver who went up to a darkened building at 2.30 in the morning.

But I had seen too many people trapped in a life of poverty who depended on the cab as their only means of transportation. Unless a situation had a real whiff of danger, I always went to the door to find the passenger. It might, I reasoned, be someone who needs my assistance. Would I not want a driver to do the same if my mother or father had called for a cab?

So, I walked to the door and knocked.

'Just a minute,' answered a frail and elderly voice. I could hear the sound of something being dragged across the floor. After a long pause, the door opened. A small woman somewhere in her 80s stood before me. She was wearing a print dress and a pillbox hat with a veil pinned on it as you might see in a costume shop or a Goodwill store or in a 1940s movie. By her side was a small nylon suitcase. The sound had been her dragging it across the floor.

The apartment looked as if no one had lived in it for years. All the furniture was covered with sheets. There were no clocks on the walls, no knick-knacks or utensils on the counters. In the corner was a cardboard box filled with photos and glassware.

'Would you carry my bag out to the car?' she said. 'I'd like a few moments alone. Then, if you could come back and help me? I'm not very strong.'

I took the suitcase to the cab and then returned to assist the woman. She took my arm, and we walked slowly toward the curb. She kept thanking me for my kindness.

'It's nothing,' I told her. 'I just try to treat my passengers the way I would want my mother treated.'

'Oh, you're such a good boy,' she said. Her praise and appreciation were almost embarrassing.

When we got in the cab, she gave me an address, and then asked, 'Could you drive through downtown?'

'It's not the shortest way,' I answered.

'Oh, I don't mind,' she said. 'I'm in no hurry. I'm on my way to a hospice.'

I looked in the rearview mirror. Her eyes were glistening.

'I don't have any family left,' she continued. 'The doctor says I should go there. He says I don't have very long.'

I quietly reached over and shut off the meter. 'What route would you like me to go?' I asked.

For the next two hours, we drove through the city. She showed me the building where she had once worked as an elevator operator. We drove through the neighbourhood where she and her husband had lived when they had first been married. She had me pull up in front of a furniture warehouse that had once been a ballroom where she had gone dancing as a girl. Sometimes she would have me slow in front of a particular building or corner and would sit staring into the darkness, saying nothing.

As the first hint of sun was creasing the horizon, she suddenly said, 'I'm tired. Let's go now.'

We drove in silence to the address she had given me. It was a low building, like a small convalescent home, with a driveway that passed under a portico. Two orderlies came out of the cab as soon as we pulled up. Without waiting for me, they opened the door and began assisting the woman. They were solicitous and intent, watching her every move. They must have been expecting her; perhaps she had phoned them right before we left.

I opened the trunk and took the small suitcase up to the door. The woman was already seated in a wheelchair. 'How much do I owe you?' she asked, reaching into her purse.

'Nothing,' I said. 'You have to make a living,' she answered.

'There are other passengers,' I responded. Almost without thinking, I bent and gave her a hug. She held on to me tightly.

'You gave an old woman a little moment of joy,' she said. 'Thank you.'

There was nothing more to say.

I squeezed her hand once, then walked out into the dim morning light. Behind me, I could hear the door shut. It was the sound of the closing of a life.

I did not pick up any more passengers that shift. I drove aimlessly, lost in thought. For the remainder of that day, I could hardly talk.

What if that woman had gotten an angry driver, or one who was impatient to end his shift? What if I had refused to take the run, or had honked once, then driven away? What if I had been in a foul mood and had refused to engage the woman in conversation? How many other moments like that had I missed or failed to grasp?

We are so conditioned to think that our lives revolve around great moments. But great moments often catch us unawares.

When that woman hugged me and said that I had brought her a moment of joy, it was possible to believe that I had been placed on earth for the sole purpose of providing her with that last ride. I do not think that I have ever done anything in my life that was any more important.

Welcome to Week Seven

BUILDING ON THE art of presence, imagine you open a door and walk directly into your next strength: patience. Cultivating patience is for many of us the most challenging of all strengths, whether you are waiting in a queue at the supermarket, or for results from a health scan, or lying in bed chasing sleep. Nature instinctively radiates patience, as Elizabeth Barrett Browning's poignant poem illustrates.

Now that you are rooted in presence, you will have the awareness to recognise the tense energy that impatience brings into your body and mind. Once you recognise it, you have a choice to build on it or to let it go.

Impatience is a block, not only to sleep, but to living fully and loving yourself and others.

The impatient mind misses opportunities to act with courage and generosity towards oneself and others. When you delay instant gratification and persevere through obstacles you will be wide awake during the day and deeply asleep at night.

✦ ✦ ✦

How Patient Are You?

IF SOMEONE ASKS if you are a patient person, what do you say? Most people will say they are not. In fact, people regularly affirm, 'I have no patience.' Why is this? It is unlikely someone would say, 'I have no kindness,' and yet patience and kindness are so interlinked, as the above story illustrates.

Admitting impatience is not just socially acceptable – people bond over their frustrations of waiting in queues, the hassle of delayed flights and how annoying it is when their partner repeats themselves. Observe the world and you will see this dissatisfaction manifest everywhere and, in particular, anytime a person is asked to wait. Considering that you are likely to spend an estimated total of six months of your life queuing for one thing or another, it is worth cultivating a calmer disposition towards this inevitable fate.

Patience is one of the most admirable traits in other people, and yet most of us struggle to grow it in ourselves.

This is hardly surprising because the etymology of the word is 'pati', which in Latin means to suffer, endure and bear. Waiting, for many people, is akin to suffering. We want results quickly and struggle to delay gratification. In a society in which speed equates to success, impatience can even be rewarded; for example, the manager in the company who puts pressure on their team to meet unrealistic deadlines or targets. In my clinical experience, impatience and a desire to be 'fixed quickly' is one of the biggest blocks to achieving and sustaining positive mental health. It is virtually impossible to help an anxious person to feel calmer when they are consumed with a sense of urgency. The faster things become, the less patience we have as a collective energy.

The study of patience is relatively new in psychology and neuroscience. What we do know is that it is a skill closely linked to mindfulness and that it can be learned. The benefits of practising patience include:

✦ An increase in positive emotions.

✦ Higher levels of self-esteem.

✦ Closer relationships.

✦ Regulated behaviours.

✦ Successfully pursuing goals and dreams.

A 2012 study published in the *Journal of Positive Psychology*, conducted by lead researcher and psychologist in this area Sarah A. Schnitker, defines patience as 'the propensity to wait calmly in the face of frustration or adversity'.[77]

Schnitker has developed a 3-Factor Patience Scale that falls into the following categories: interpersonal patience, life hardship patience and daily hassles patience.

Take this questionnaire now and test your own patience. Answer as honestly as you can and be patient as you work out your scores!

3-FACTOR PATIENCE SCALE QUESTIONNAIRE

For each of the statements below, please indicate how much the statement is like/unlike you.

1 = Not like me at all
2 = Unlike me
3 = Neutral
4 = Like me
5 = Very much like me

1 My friends would say I'm a very patient friend.

2 I am able to wait out tough times.

3 Although they're annoying, I don't get too upset when stuck in traffic jams.

4 I am patient with other people.

5 I find it pretty easy to be patient with a difficult life problem or illness.

6 In general, waiting in lines does not bother me.

7 I find it easy to be patient with my close friends and family.

8 I am patient during life's hardships.

9 When someone is having difficulty learning something new, I will be able to help them without getting frustrated or annoyed.

10 I don't get annoyed at red lights.

11 I find it easy to be patient with people.

Add up your results in the three following categories that define different aspects of patience.

✦ Factor 1 – Interpersonal patience: Questions 1, 4, 7, 9, 11

✦ Factor 2 – Life hardship patience: Questions 2, 5, 8

✦ Factor 3 – Daily hassles patience: Questions 3, 6, 10

The higher the score in each category, the higher the level of patience you have. Please note that there are five questions on interpersonal patience and only three in the remaining two categories, life hardship and daily hassles, so take this into consideration when adding up your results.

You may be surprised to learn you are more patient in some areas compared to others; for example, getting stuck in a traffic jam doesn't irritate you, but being patient with a family member who always repeats themselves causes you to get irritated quickly.

INTERPERSONAL PATIENCE

Often, we are most impatient with those closest to us. A busy mind is one that hurries others along, and the tempo of your thoughts has a direct correlation to your level of patience. If your mind is always in planning mode, you will find it much more difficult to connect with and wait for the people you love.

Our partners, our children and our parents are the people most likely to experience our harsher voice, our irritability and our desire that they operate life at the same speed as us. The reason being, of course, that we feel safest with them. Zen Buddhist monk Thich Nhat Hanh said that if you treat your partner as a guest in your home, you will cultivate love and patience. In his book *How to Love* he said, 'There's a tradition in Asia of treating your partner with the respect you would accord a guest. This is true even if you have been with your loved one for a long time. The other person always deserves your full respect. Reverence is the nature of our love.'

To help you cultivate this, consider who is the most patient person you know. How do you feel in their presence? For many of us, and for the reasons outlined above, it is not the people we spend most of our time with. It is often a grandparent, a friend or an older sibling. This was certainly true for me. My grandmother Olive and my great-aunt Lally (her sister), to whom this book is dedicated, exuded patience. A few months ago, I was out for lunch with my dad, and I asked him to tell me more about his own grandmother. I wanted to know more about the woman who had given birth to two women who have shaped my life with so much love.

My father told me he recalled his grandmother as someone who was affectionate and loving but who, unfortunately, got dementia when he was a child. He said she would be sitting in her own living room and all of a sudden she would say, 'We have the same curtains at home, I want to go home now.' My great-aunt Lally, who was her prime carer, would say, 'OK, then let's go home.' She would get her mother's coat and bag and they would leave by the back entrance of the house, get into the car and drive around the block. Lally would then park, and they would enter through the front door. This is interpersonal patience personified.

One of the ways I work on improving my own patience is to bring the energy of Auntie Lally to mind and allow her to guide me. You can do the same. Bring your patient person to mind when you feel irritation arising and ask yourself, 'What would they say or do?' Sometimes it is being proactive and sometimes it is simply remaining silent.

Patience is not passive. When it comes to practising patience with your loved ones it is important not to fall into pretending everything is fine, if it is not. Patience is not about being perfect and devoid of frustration. Suppressing your irritation in order to be more patient can easily leak into passive aggressiveness. Patience needs to be genuine and heartfelt. Be courageous and mindfully explain how you feel when you feel impatient. For example, if every morning you wake up early to carve out quiet time for yourself to meditate or journal, but your family now also decides to wake up and look for your attention, you need to explain calmly that this solo time is yours. Set a boundary for when you will be back 'on duty' again! This is harder, of course, with young children, especially if you are a single parent.

It is helpful to think of patience as a process rather than a product.

Explaining to your loved ones when you feel your patience is thin is also very helpful. Simply state that you are finding it hard to remain calm; perhaps you had a long day and are feeling overwhelmed. Context is essential, and remember, patience is not independent of proactivity. You can stand up for yourself, set boundaries and be an active agent of change. Calmly encourage change from a place of equanimity and balance. Emotional states are contagious and the more patient you become the more you will inspire those around you to do the same.

LIFE HARDSHIP PATIENCE

Many people, understandably, struggle with patience when they receive a serious health diagnosis such as cancer, or have an accident that requires them to be out of action for months if not years. When life as you know it is turned upside down, your patience will be tested.

> **Patient becomes both a verb and a noun when your health is compromised.**

It is often in these hard times that your sleep is also disturbed by both physical and psychological pain. From a medical perspective, 'the pill for every ill' is an example of people not wanting to wait or take the time to heal. Medication has a hugely significant role to play in many illnesses, yet it can only ever be part of the solution – and in some cases, it can cause more harm than good. The idea that a pill will fix you, whether it is a sleeping pill or a cure for obesity, devalues the power of your mind and distracts from lifestyle interventions that can prevent many non-communicable diseases arising in the first place.

If you find your health compromised, perspective and acknowledging the most minuscule steps of progress will help significantly. Letting go of the person you were in terms of fitness and activity levels will help you to embrace your life now rather than what it once was. Acceptance of a new reality is not easy and requires a lot of time and tears. Living alongside chronic health conditions may not be ideal, but it is possible. If you stay stuck in resistance to reality, you will become stagnant, and this is true in all areas of your life. Becoming emotionally agile and tolerating uncertainty is essential, whether you are navigating an illness, trying to get pregnant or searching for a new house.

DAILY HASSLES PATIENCE

Letting go of minor irritations in life, and there are many, for example heavy traffic when you are late, being put on hold by your bank for hours, rain on the day of your summer barbecue, misplacing your keys or your glasses again, and the list goes on ... all of these hassles are what Michael Singer, author of the bestselling book *The Untethered Soul*, refers to as 'the low-hanging fruit'.

The low-hanging fruit provides material to practise the art of letting go of events, people and circumstances out of your control. Smiling in the rain on your holiday, breathing deeply when you forget your phone in a hotel, letting go of the mess in your children's or teenagers' bedrooms.

> **Choosing to cultivate patience for these minor but multiple daily stressors is doing the fieldwork for when bigger adversities come your way.**

It is so important to cleanse and clear emotionally as you go through your day. When you feel irritation and impatience arise, recognise them and ask yourself why you are getting frustrated. Ask yourself, is this within or outside my control? Many daily hassles are out of your control. For example, you do not choose to have a delayed flight, and yet you are not in a position to change it. Viewing these moments as opportunities to practise patience is immensely empowering. You will begin to embrace the moments you are asked to wait as windows of time when you are blessed to be and not to do.

The red light becomes your friend, the long line in the supermarket is a chance to press 'Pause' and observe the world. You will be amazed at what you witness when frustration with reality dissipates. Each time you do this in your day, you are setting the scene for a peaceful mind, which is the third and most crucial strength for sleep.

PATIENCE TO REALISE YOUR DREAMS

Cultivating patience is not only beneficial for nurturing closer bonds with people and dealing with daily or more difficult hardships; it is also incredibly powerful to help you succeed in setting and maintaining goals. Delaying gratification is imperative if, for example, you want to start a business, write a book, pass exams, return to third-level education, improve your golf swing, strengthen your tennis serve or perfect your downward dog in yoga. For many of these pursuits, it is going to take years before you see concrete results.

The most well-known study on the area of delayed gratification is the 1972 Stanford Marshmallow Experiment.[78] Psychologist Walter Mischel and his colleagues invited four-year-olds into their lab and placed a tempting marshmallow in front of them. The children were given a choice: they were told they could either eat the sweet immediately or wait 15 minutes. If the sweet remained untouched, they would be given an extra marshmallow as a reward. Fifteen minutes is a big ask for most adults to wait for their morning coffee, never mind a young child in a room alone.

The footage of the children shows a range of reactions, from the ones who grabbed the sweet as soon as the adult left the room to the conflicted child who wriggled around before eventually succumbing to temptation. It was a minority of kids who were able to sit it out and received their reward of the second sweet. The follow-up research showed that the patient children, when they reached adolescence, displayed higher levels of social, emotional and academic intelligence, and they were less likely to abuse substances or be obese.[79] This study has been replicated numerous times with varying results.

How do you think you would have performed in such a study at four years of age? Of course, you will never know, but it is never too late to train yourself to be more patient. You will discover what an act of love it is to be the person who waits. To hold the door open, to let someone go in front of you at the supermarket or in traffic, to slowly build on your dreams, to be patient if you enter a lighter phase of sleep and to know that sleep will return when it is ready.

One of the key tenets for cultivating patience is to bring an altruistic component to your motivation to practice it. For example, your ageing mother tells you the same story for the tenth time, your young child is having a temper tantrum for no fathomable reason or your teenager takes their frustrations out on you. Seeing beyond people's behaviour and putting it into the context of their lives and challenges will help you to help them. Focus on the loving energy you give rather than the behaviour that used to cause you irritation.

PATIENCE FOR SLEEP

Taking patience to bed with you will help you to manage the nights when you are on higher alert, for example when you are travelling early the next morning, or you have a big presentation that you wish to perform well at. Patience allows you to be gentle with yourself and to take extra time to unwind in your bedtime routine. You have faith that your sleep will return to its optimum state very soon. If you wake up in a lighter stage of sleep, patience is again helpful. You are not forcing or rushing the process of letting go. You simply allow it to happen. The energy of patience is reinforced in your hypnotherapy audios. All it requires is your commitment to listen. This week's habit (taking time to rest every day in the middle of your day) is another opportunity to practise patience; resting and napping during your day is a rehearsal for bedtime. You are training your mind and body to let go and surrender to rest, which is the first step to sleep.

Reflective Journaling Prompts

✦ How do you feel when you are with a patient person?

✦ When in your life have you delayed gratification? Has it paid off?

✦ Write down the daily triggers that cause you to feel impatient.

✦ ✦ ✦

Positive Practice

✦ In the moments when you find yourself forced to wait, rather than adding to the frustration (recall the two arrows), practise gratitude for the opportunity to pick the low-hanging fruit. You are practising patience for the times in your life when you will need it most.

✦ If you drive, can you consciously choose to look for at least one opportunity on each journey to let another car out in front of you? Then start to increase this to three. It becomes a game, where you are actually seeking opportunities to wait and also helping others.

✦ ✦ ✦

Affirmations to Repeat

✦ 'I am a patient person.'

✦ 'Love motivates me to wait for others.'

✦ 'I welcome opportunities to wait.'

Build Your Sleep Well Habits

CONTINUE WITH THE habits you've formed in the previous weeks:

✦ Habit One: You go to sleep and wake up at roughly the same time every day.

✦ Habit Two: You have a 'blissful hour' bedtime routine.

✦ Habit Three: You move your body.

✦ Habit Four: You reduce your alcohol and caffeine intake.

✦ Habit Five: You optimise your light and temperature exposure.

✦ Habit Six: You eat mindfully and at regular times.

HABIT SEVEN

Take Time to Rest Every Day in The Middle of Your Day

> The time to relax is when you don't have time for it.
>
> SYDNEY J. HARRIS

TO NAP OR NOT?

As I mentioned before, taking a rest or short sleep in the day takes patience. The default is to think you don't have time to rest. In fact, please do bear in mind the opposite is true: you don't have time *not* to rest. Even if your 'rest' is distilled into closing your eyes and taking seven deep breaths on a busy day, it is better than no rest at all. When you close your eyes and breathe deeply you are acknowledging the need to connect to your inner world. You are saying to part of you that is tired, *I see you, I hear you and I want to help.*

As a young child, I lived on the Greek island of Paros, and one of the lifestyle habits that I brought home with me was the siesta, the time of day when, due to the heat of the sun, the Greek people retreat inside to sleep and/or rest. Ikaria, another Greek island, known as 'the island where people forget to die', is one of the five 'Blue Zones' in the world. The Blue Zones are geographical pockets dotted all over the world that have a significantly higher than average number of centenarians (people aged over 100). Not only do Ikarians live longer, but they also have lower rates of cancer and heart disease.[80] They are less prone to dementia and tend to remain physically and sexually active deep into their 90s.

One in-depth study over six years on a population of 24,000 Greek adults showed that regular napping reduced the risk of heart disease by almost 40 per cent. It was shown that this figure was increased in people who worked as opposed to those who were unemployed. It appears that a mid-afternoon rest can offset the stress of work.[81]

The science shows that 'strategic napping' needs to be early after lunch and short. If you over-nap, you enter into deep sleep, and this is always much more difficult to wake from. A maximum of 30 minutes before 2.30 p.m. is ideal.

If you are already a napper, then great. If you're not, and you don't feel the need to take one (as in, you are not tired), then you don't need to start. Still, it is imperative you take some time to rest and connect to yourself halfway through your day.

The seven-minute rest ritual included in this programme is designed to be a realistic tool for you to do at least once a day. I know that many people are not in a position to take a full rest during their working week. It is a privilege, but it is not a luxury. I encourage you to find a way to take just seven minutes for yourself. You don't have to be lying down to do the shavasana (if you can, do!). Sitting at your desk or on a train or bus with earphones is still very effective.

Deep relaxation is a rehearsal period for when you go to bed and let go.

Andrew Huberman coined the phrase non-sleep deep rest (NSDR) and makes sure he rests or naps most days. The use of hypnosis or a yoga nidra script (which is a guided visualisation and progressive body relaxation) are both effective ways to activate your parasympathetic nervous system and boost your energy levels. The more you train yourself to relax during the day, the easier it is for you to unwind in your blissful hour. Remember that you can also use night-time audio as a guided nap and rehearsal for sleep.

After a period of activity, you need to rest your body and mind. When you take the time to rest, you are also taking the time to connect to yourself on an emotional level. You are checking in with your internal state and if for any reason you are not OK, then you are in a position to embrace what is going on before you get into bed that night.

The more you connect to your inner world during the day, the less overwhelming life is when you close your eyes at night. You are also less likely to reawaken due to unexplained angst.

A Story of Surrendering to Sleep

The shavasana, also known as the death pose or corpse pose in yoga, is an extremely effective way to practise a deep rest in a short period of time. Included in this programme is the seven-minute rest ritual recorded by one of the best yoga teachers I have, Rohan Hennessy.

Rohan began teaching iyengar yoga (an emphasis on detail, precision and alignment) in 2000 before moving towards vinyasa. His classes are strong and slow, challenging yet also calming. He believes the asana (pose) should adapt to suit the body instead of vice versa.

Rohan's shavasana, which is practised at the end of a class to rest the body entirely after movement, is the best I've ever had, and I had to share it with you. You will really benefit from it, as so many of his students do.

When I met Rohan to discuss his involvement in the book, he told me the following story about his own sleep. Perhaps you recognise parts of yourself or others you love in it.

My sleep issues probably began at a very young age as I have many childhood memories of not wanting to go to bed. I think that I felt that I was missing out on something. My parents would sometimes have friends over quite late, and I was often allowed to stay up, and I'm sure this was part of it. My dad was usually awake until the early hours most nights too. As a teenager, I was up late most nights and slept late whenever I could. When I left home at 19, I was playing music for a living and had no set routine. I would sometimes be awake all night and through the next day. I had never taken cocaine, ecstasy, speed or anything like that so that wasn't the issue.

I levelled out a bit in my twenties but still didn't like going to bed early and struggled with early mornings. In my thirties, it got worse, and my circadian rhythm was all over the place. I would be awake progressively later night by night, to the point where I was going to work in the morning on zero sleep and collapsing into afternoon naps. It would reset every few months (when I was exhausted) and I would get a week or so of good nights' sleep but then it would slip later and later until it was upside down again.

I was used to it and used to struggle through it. I never went to see anyone about it, but it was getting harder as the years went by, so I was considering looking for help. But then almost all of a sudden, it began to regulate. I'm not sure when exactly, sometime over the past 12–18 months, I think.

I still like to stay up a little later, but I get tired at a reasonable hour every night and feel content going to bed. I usually wake up early but sometimes also enjoy a lie-in. It honestly feels like a weight that I was carrying for years and had been growing heavier with time has been lifted. It's amazing, really!

I think there are several things that contributed to this. Discipline, job satisfaction, staying active, etc. But there must be more to it as well. At various points over the years, I felt afraid that I might die in my sleep. I found a conversation we recently had interesting, in which we discussed sleep being a mini death each night. Maybe we need to learn to let go, to surrender to sleep, to the idea of this mini death, to the mystery of being alive and eventually to death itself and whatever that may bring.

What this Looks Like for Me

I nap or rest on the days my schedule allows it. It can be for as much as 30 minutes or sometimes only 10. Often, I listen to a hypnotherapy audio. Other times, I just close my eyes and doze. I've been known to nap in busy places, for example under the statue of David in Florence, which was a nice view! If I'm out and about and I can, I will rest in my car or find a spot to sit down where I can use my headphones and drift for a while. If this is not possible, I will close my eyes and take seven deep belly breaths as a way of acknowledging the need to retreat within and connect to myself. Sometimes, I read a spiritual book just after the rest to allow the teachings to soak in when I am still a little drowsy, which is an ideal window for neuroplastic change. If I am dealing with a challenge in my life, I may do some journaling, so that I am not leaving my emotions to build up before bed.

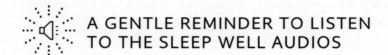

A GENTLE REMINDER TO LISTEN TO THE SLEEP WELL AUDIOS

You can access these audios for FREE with the passcode ISLEEPWELL on www.thepositivehabit.com.

Please remember to listen to the instructions for listening to guarantee maximum benefits.

MORNING MEDITATION

Please listen each morning to 'Start Your Day in Stillness – Intention-Setting Morning Meditation' to slow down your thoughts, before the day commences.

Please listen to 'Seven-Minute Rest Ritual' each afternoon and/
or evening.

NIGHT-TIME HYPNOTHERAPY – WEEK SEVEN: HABIT SEVEN
This is the most important track to listen to. Each week there
are new subconscious suggestions to help to reinforce the
corresponding weekly habit and the following key insights.

To Get Back to Sleep if You Wake Up
You can listen to your night-time audio again, if necessary, but
with time you will not need to do this. The Sleep Well Formula
(Breathe + Imagine + Experience = Faith) which you are learning
on a subconscious level every time you listen to your weekly audios
will become automatic. Please also listen to the '4, 7, 8 Breathing'
audio and train yourself to do this in the middle of the night
should you awaken.

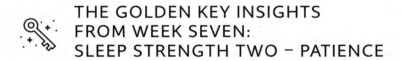

THE GOLDEN KEY INSIGHTS FROM WEEK SEVEN: SLEEP STRENGTH TWO – PATIENCE

✦ Cultivating patience is for many of us the most challenging strength
to develop. Impatience is the biggest block to sleeping well and
living fully.

✦ This is hardly surprising because the etymology of the word is 'pati',
which in Latin means to suffer, endure and bear. Waiting, for many,
is akin to suffering. We want results quickly and struggle to delay
gratification. Be gentle with yourself when you are impatient.

- The good news is that patience is a skill closely linked to mindfulness and that it can be learned. The benefits of practising patience include an increase in positive emotions, higher levels of self-esteem, closer relationships, regulated behaviours and successfully pursuing goals and dreams.

- Recall which type of patience you find most challenging: interpersonal patience, life hardship patience or daily hassles patience.

- This week's habit, 'Take time to rest every day in the middle of your day', is another opportunity to practise patience. Resting and napping during your day is a rehearsal for bedtime. You are training your mind and body to let go and surrender to rest, which is the first step to sleep.

To maximise the benefits of this programme, I encourage you not to begin reading Week Eight until you have listened to the 'Week Seven: Habit Seven' night-time audio for a minimum of seven nights in total.

You are making wonderful progress, and patience is the strength that you will need to keep returning to. I know I do! It really helps on the nights when your sleep is broken or interrupted by circumstances out of your control.

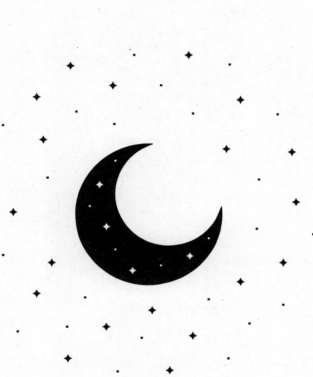

SLEEP
STRENGTH
THREE - PEACE

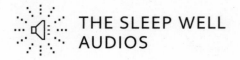

THE SLEEP WELL AUDIOS

All audios are available to download on www.thepositivehabit.com with the password ISLEEPWELL.

✦ **Tonight, please start listening to 'Week Eight: Habit Eight' of the Sleep Well audios. Please listen to this audio for a minimum of seven nights.**

✦ **Please also continue to listen to your morning meditation and your rest ritual hypnotherapy tracks each day.**

✦ ✦ ✦

Measure Your Sleep

BEFORE YOU BEGIN Week Eight of the Sleep Well Programme, please take a moment to rate your sleep. On a scale of 0 to 10, how well have you slept in the last week? (0 is 'terribly' and 10 is 'very well'.) Please use the image on the opposite page to mark where you feel you are on this scale.

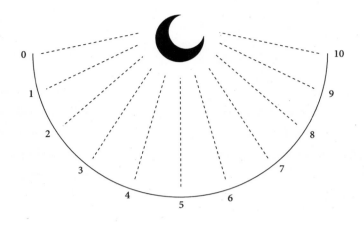

✦ ✦ ✦

A Poem to Fall Asleep With

Peace

Peace flows into me
As the tide to the pool by the shore;
It is mine forevermore,
It ebbs not back like the sea.
I am the pool of blue
That worships the vivid sky;
My hopes were heaven-high,
They are all fulfilled in you.
I am the pool of gold
When sunset burns and dies,
You are my deepening skies,
Give me your stars to hold.

SARA TEASDALE, 1884–1933

Welcome to Week Eight

THE NEXT STRENGTH that you are welcoming into your bed and life is peace. After presence and patience, its soft light will help you to drift to sleep at night and help you to be content with what you have and who you are. A good sleeper, like you, requires a peaceful mind, a light consciousness and the faith that sleep is a gift from nature that is effortless to welcome.

✦ ✦ ✦

A Story to Fall Asleep With

THE FOLLOWING STORY is based on a client case study. I have changed any identifying factors to protect the person's anonymity.

Gary always wanted more. More money, more power, more success, more kids, more holidays, more work. Once he had more, he said, he would be at peace. Once he had enough, he would sleep properly and take better care of himself.

Gary was from Scotland and grew up in an ashram (a spiritual community) with his parents, who were part of a cult. This cult asked the family to donate all their worldly possessions to the community, including selling their family home. The leader of the community had a godlike status and ruled his kingdom with hypocrisy and fear.

Gary and his younger brother were taught wonderful spiritual teachings, but only in theory. The reality they witnessed was the opposite. Every day, they saw the power struggle among the adults in the community as they vied for their leader's attention. Gary's parents argued all the time and were the opposite of calm, and the ashram was a place of chaos and confusion. Gary and his brother saw their parents tear each other apart: the financial stress of giving away everything they owned created havoc.

When I met Gary he was in a precarious position; he was working 12-hour days Monday to Friday and at weekends; he was eating junk food and getting no exercise; and his sleep was so poor that some nights he wasn't sure if he had slept at all. Gary was on the cusp of burnout.

His parents had now left the community and were living in poverty, and were constantly asking him for money. On the plus side, he was happily married to an Irish woman and had two young children who he adored. He had built a highly successful career as an investment banker and was constantly promoted and headhunted. However, he rarely saw his children; he was sleeping an average of five hours a night and he was intelligent enough to know that this situation was not tenable. Gary had many financial fears. No matter how much his salary was, it was never enough; he feared that it could all be taken away from him. Of course, knowing his story, you can see why.

Through our work, Gary began to realise it wasn't money that was never enough, but how he felt about himself. His parents had always been pursuing the approval of their guru and he had felt insignificant, forgotten about and left to play alone for hours. When I compassionately pointed out that things were no different today, that he too was seeking approval from his 'corporate master' and his own children were missing out, he slowly began to wake up to the reality of his situation.

Gary lacked inner peace and understandably rejected a meditation practice or any spiritual teachings. We worked together to help him revisit many of the positive learnings that he had been exposed to as a child. He had a wealth of knowledge that just needed to be put into practice. During a hypnotherapy session, a long-forgotten memory came back to Gary. He recalled one day back in the ashram when he was roughly seven years old, when a young woman (another member of the community) came to his rescue while his parents were having one of their frequent and terrifying arguments.

She took his hand and asked him to close his eyes and to put his two fingers in his ears to help tune out the sound of his parents tearing each other apart. She asked him what he could see.

'Nothing,' he said.

She asked him what he could hear.

'Nothing,' he repeated.

'What does nothing feel like?' she asked.

'Nice,' he replied.

'That "nothing" is your peace,' she told him. **'No matter what happened in your life, the peace you seek is within you.'**

Nobody can take your 'nothing' away from you. Through our work, 'peace is within me' became Gary's mantra. As an adult, he could see that the nothing he described as a child was everything he ever needed.

Gary was dedicated to listening to the night-time hypnotherapy audios and his sleep improved quickly. Once his sleep was better, Gary had the energy and the clarity to set healthy boundaries in his life. At work, he told his boss he would be offline from 5.30 p.m. every day and at weekends. When he went on holiday, he went on holiday. He began to spend more time with his children. He stopped sending money to his parents, as they were both still young enough to seek basic employment, which they did. Gary's progress was not overnight, and to this day a feeling of not being good enough can emerge. However, he knows that being content with who he is and not what he has is the route to a peaceful mind.

Peace is Contentment

WHAT DOES CONTENTMENT mean to you? More important, what does it feel like? Like many words that describe emotions and feelings, interpretations can vary. Personally, contentment is pure peace with what is here and now. No striving or yearning for more is necessary.

This moment is enough, I have enough, my life is enough, I am enough.

This full feeling is naturally restful and conducive to sleep. A recent study published in *Frontiers in Psychology* called 'A time to sleep well and be contented: time perspective, sleep quality, and life satisfaction' found that good quality sleep and feelings of contentment are indeed interlinked.[82]

Time perspective is how you view your past, present and future, either through a negative or a positive lens. The study found that individuals who have a positive time perspective have higher levels of life satisfaction and therefore better sleep quality.

THE PEACE OF MIND SCALE

The following scale was published in the *Journal of Happiness Studies* in a research paper entitled 'The Construct and Measurement of Peace of Mind'.[83]

How often do you feel internal peace and ease in your daily life?

Use the following scale to indicate your response.

1 = Not at all
2 = Some of the time
3 = Often
4 = Most of the time
5 = All the time

Questions

1 My mind is free and at ease.

2 I feel content and comfortable with myself in daily life.

3 My lifestyle gives me feelings of peace and stability.

4 I have peace and harmony in my mind.

5 The way I live brings me feelings of peace and comfort.

The highest score you can get **overall** is 25. The higher your overall score, the more peace of mind and harmony you feel.

A feeling of peace, like patience, is not something that comes easily for many people. Resistance to being fully satisfied with, first, what you have and, second and more fundamentally, who you are is common. The fear that if you settle you will stagnate is one that stops many people from enjoying the benefits of living a peaceful life. Contentment is not complacency; inner peace is the springboard for continued success and happiness.

On a subconscious level, if you are content with what you have materially and financially, this can be deemed a threat. Your hunter/gatherer brain is primed to seek more even when you consciously know you have enough. There is a fear that if you take it easy your security could all be taken away. This fear creates a disconnect from the reality, which is that many of us have more than enough. If you are blessed, like I am, to have a warm bed to sleep in each night in a safe place, then you can count yourself as privileged beyond measure. According to a report by the United Nations, an estimated 1.6 billion people worldwide were living in inadequate housing or homelessness as of 2020. This statistic includes people living in slums or in unsafe dwellings and since Covid-19 the number has unfortunately risen. Shelter is a human right, and people who do not have shelter have every reason to strive for more.

While it is worth being aware of and grateful for your privilege, if you have it, it is not helpful to compare yourself to those less well-off. When you do this, it often elicits feelings of guilt, and this is not a useful energy for you to sleep well or to contribute to humanity. People in need do not need pity; they require proactivity.

Transform feelings of guilt into compassionate action. For example, if you are well rested you are in a physical state of abundance and in a position to actually help people in need. You can share the energy you garner from your good night's sleep to volunteer in a shelter or simply take the time to stop and say hello to a homeless person. Your best-slept self seizes opportunities to help others.

> **The most valuable commodity you have is your energy and when you have an abundance it overflows into those who need it most.**

THE MYTH OF MORE

The 'hedonic treadmill' is the dysfunctional belief that having more will make you happier. This psychological condition is so common, we don't even question it. It is one of the prime blocks to peace. A seminal study carried out in 1978 sought to question this.[84] The researchers examined the relationship between income levels and overall levels of happiness. They looked at three groups of individuals: lottery winners, paralysed accident victims and a control group of individuals who had not experienced any significant positive or negative life events.

The researchers found that both the lottery winners and the paralysed accident victims experienced a boost or decline in happiness respectively after the major event, but over time their levels of happiness returned to their baseline levels. The control group, on the other hand, showed no significant change in happiness over time. This research reinforces the idea that in order to feel peace you must seek it within and not in your external world.

Subjective peace and well-being are determined by both nature and nurture. The question of how much is attributed to either remains unanswered, with some studies claiming genetics are responsible for as much as 44 per cent and others saying it is a mere 10 per cent. While the science is unclear, we know through the study of neuroplasticity that that you can consciously create a peaceful state of mind. To do this, it is essential to know on a deep level that peace is not caused by anything external.

Practising non-attachment, not only to your possessions but also to the external outcomes in your life, ensures that peace is always present. It does not mean that you do not own beautiful things; in fact, it is the contrary – beautiful things do not own you. If you lose them, you lose them. If it is time to give them away, it is time to give them away. A few years ago, my husband and I sold the little French home that we had had for 10 years, nestled in a small village in the vineyards. It is a place where time stands still and peace is the currency of the land. Our son was six months old when we first went. We watched him grow there each summer. We had collected a decade of possessions, and many had great sentimental value. When we made the decision to sell the home, we gave all the contents away. Every single thing. It was liberating. The reality, though, is that we gave nothing of value away: the house and the memories live in each of us, and the peace from that time guides us today.

The ability to enjoy what you have in the now allows you to realise that your possessions, your home, and your physical appearance are all transient. You make the most of what you have, and then you let it go.

Inner peace does not mean you do not aspire to great things. You do aspire to improve your life and others' lives, but the outcome, whether it is positive or not what you had hoped, does not dictate the peace of your being. You are at peace regardless. The contented person approaches life from a place that is full and not lacking, and they make choices in line with their values rather than a fear of not having or being enough. As we saw in Gary's story, often underneath the fear of not having enough is the fear of not being enough.

The universal negative and self-limiting belief of 'I am not good enough' is one that plagues people regardless of age and cultural background.

THE AUTHENTIC AND PEACEFUL SELF

The roots of this belief are often born in childhood and adolescence. When a child feels that love is conditional, they will begin to shape themselves according to what they think is acceptable to their parents and other figures of authority. The authentic self is shut down and the conditioned self is born. The conditioned self is exactly that – a personality that is shaped by its environment and one that relies on meeting certain criteria to feel that the person is loved. For example, if you grew up in a house that valued productivity and hard work and resting or relaxing was seen as lazy, you may feel that you are not enough unless you are achieving or working.

Donald Winnicott was a British paediatrician and psychoanalyst who contributed extensively to the field of child development and psychoanalytic theory. He once said, 'It is a joy to be hidden, and a disaster never to be found.' Take a moment to consider what this quote means to you. At first glance, for many, it appears to be a paradox; however, it is saying that a child needs the liberty of their own private world and at the same time to know that there is an adult who understands and loves this authentic part of them.

Winnicott spoke about how 'the false self' is born in childhood when a child does not feel accepted for who they are but rather as a construct that suits the parent. For example, a child who is obedient not because they choose to be but rather because they are rewarded for doing what they are told. The false self then becomes a façade, and this creates a block to the authentic self. This block can create much confusion and psychological distress later in life. For example, the build-up of suppressed emotion that was never voiced turns into self-loathing and low self-esteem.

It can be hard to be at peace with who you are if as a child you felt invisible.

Carl Jung's aforementioned 'shadow self' is connected to Winnicott's 'false self' in that in order to survive, a part of you is hidden. This can lead to misdirected internalised shame. For example, if your mother suffered from postnatal depression and was unable to bond with you, it is possible that you internalised this lack of connection as somehow your fault and a feeling of being unworthy emerged.

This is just one example and there are countless others. Childhood trauma does not have to be a major event or tragedy within the family; it is often a slow and subtle build-up of what is unsaid and unseen that causes a child to question their value.

Brené Brown is a research professor at the University of Houston and a leading voice in the fields of shame, vulnerability and self-esteem. She has emphasised the need for people to build self-compassion as a tool to combat the inner voice that erodes inner peace. Studies have shown that people who have high levels of self-compassion have lower levels of anxiety and depression.[85]

I truly hope that these insights and understandings of your conditioned self bring some clarity. No matter what the events have been in your life, or the ideas that you formed about yourself when you were a child, you deserve to be at peace in both your waking and sleeping state. When you have this 'knowing' that peace is within you, you too are free.

Peace is faith. Faith is unshakable and permanent. It induces a level of inner peace like you might have never experienced before. When you have faith, you do not question.

Faith in yourself brings a feeling of inner peace, doubt dissolves and you are centred and sleeping peacefully. Your belief in your ability to sleep at night and your ability to shine during the day are in essence the same thing: when you wake up to life, you sleep peacefully. In order to sustain a peaceful mind, you need to release limiting beliefs that you hold about yourself.

✦ ✦ ✦

Are you benefiting from a secondary gain?

MANY PEOPLE SUBCONSCIOUSLY cling to negative beliefs for underlying reasons that are not apparent to them on a conscious level. In John Boyne's magnificent novel *The Heart's Invisible Furies* he described one of his characters as 'being a martyr to the insomnia'. She would be wide awake at all hours and seemed to take a bizarre pride in this. She also liked to keep an eye on the comings and goings in her street. Her curiosity being satisfied as to 'what the neighbours were up to' is what is known in psychology as a secondary gain.

A running narrative throughout this book has been to question the stories that you have been telling yourself. At this stage in your Sleep Well journey, if for any reason you find yourself remaining resistant, it could be that the lure of a secondary gain is blocking your progress. Be mindful that this is not your fault. However, we need to unearth any possible hidden gains you may feel you are getting from remaining 'a bad sleeper'.

In my clinical experience over the years many clients who cling to an identity of being a 'hopeless case' when it comes to sleep illustrate the following secondary gains:

✦ **Attention and sympathy:** Enjoying the concern and support others offer on an ongoing basis, for example, 'How is the sleep now?', 'It must be so hard... you poor thing', 'I don't know how you cope.'

✦ **Avoidance of responsibility:** Using sleep difficulties as a way to avoid certain responsibilities or tasks, especially those perceived as challenging or stressful.

✦ **Excuse for underperformance:** Providing a ready-made excuse for underperforming at work or in other areas of life, shifting blame to the perceived inability to sleep well. (Remember, this is not intentional.)

✦ **Special treatment:** Being treated differently or receiving special considerations from others due to the perceived struggle with sleep. For example, when you go away with friends or family you need your own room.

- ✦ **Social connection:** Finding common ground with others who also struggle with sleep, leading to a sense of belonging and shared experiences.

- ✦ **External validation:** Receiving validation or reassurance from others about the severity of their sleep issues, reinforcing the identity of being a hopeless case.

- ✦ **Avoidance of certain activities:** Using sleep difficulties as a reason to avoid trying new things from a work perspective or attending social events.

- ✦ **Personal time and space:** Gaining personal time and space while others have to accommodate you or give you extra space due to the perceived struggle with sleep. For example, staying in bed longer in the mornings.

Just notice if any of these resonate with you. Once you become aware of one secondary gain or more, they can no longer control you. That is not to say that many of these gains are valid needs, for example more social connection and personal space. It is the means by which you are getting them that is not serving you.

The ARC mindfulness tool from Week Three: Your Waking Self will help you to break these associations. A bird needs two wings to fly. One wing is your mindful awareness of a secondary gain and the second wing is having compassion towards yourself. For example, if having read the above list, you are now aware that you enjoy the sympathy you get from others for being a bad sleeper, you need to offer compassion to the part of you that feeds on this sympathy. No judgement. People cling to unhealthy behaviours and dysfunctional beliefs not because they want to, but often because they feel they are protecting themselves. The reality is that secondary benefits are often a false friend and ultimately only curtail your peace of mind and capacity to sleep well.

PEACE FOR SLEEP

'May they rest in peace' is the expression often used when a person dies. Why wait until you die to rest in peace? You have every night to do this. Peace comes from stillness and silence. You have access to this 'nothingness' each night.

What bliss. What a joy it is to die to the day.
To surrender to the darkness.

It is said that many people who are given a short time to live fall in love with life and exude peace. You can see it emanate, not only from those who have a fatal illness, but also from some older people who have decided to give up suffering. They say that when death comes closer, there is a profound peace that comes with it. No more fear. The darkness within, so to speak, has been removed and therefore the literal black of the night poses no threat. It brings light, it brings peace.

I don't know how old you are, or the state of your health. I do, however, have faith in you. I know you are as capable of sleeping peacefully as anybody else. In order for you to feel this inner peace as you drift off, you need to welcome it into your day. The strengths of presence and patience will naturally invite peace to emerge. It is perhaps easier to welcome peace on a warm summer's day in a country meadow or as you gaze at a sunset or hold a smiling baby, but this same peace is always available to you. Amid the chaos and noise and the busyness of your life, there is serenity. The deeper you sleep, the more you witness the space under daytime dramas –

both those outside of you and the thoughts in your mind. In doing so, you welcome with grace the peace that awaits you each and every night. From this place, slowly, slowly, sweet slumber unfolds.

Build Your Sleep Well Habits

CONTINUE WITH THE habits you've formed in the previous weeks:

+ Habit One: You go to sleep and wake up at roughly the same time every day.

+ Habit Two: You have a 'blissful hour' bedtime routine.

+ Habit Three: You move your body.

+ Habit Four: You reduce your alcohol and caffeine intake.

+ Habit Five: You optimise light and temperature exposure.

+ Habit Six: You eat mindfully and at regular times.

+ Habit Seven: You take time to rest in the middle of the day.

HABIT EIGHT

Laugh Often and Enjoy Positive Connections

A day without laughter is a day wasted.

CHARLIE CHAPLIN

ALWAYS LEAVE THE best till last. Psychologists and neuroscientists suggest the evolutionary reason why we laugh is that it is the best non-verbal way to form social bonds, release tension and regulate emotion. It is also often the most immediate method to defuse a conflict or quell a drama.

Can you recall how much you laughed when you were a child? As a teenager?

If laughter could be measured, what percentage of your day is spent laughing now compared to then? I heard once that children laugh 300 times a day and adults a mere 17 times. This seems stark; however, when you spend time with children you certainly notice they do laugh more. There are, I am sure, a combination of reasons why this is the case. They have less responsibility, more time to spend with friends – but I believe that laughter, like sleep, is innate and we are all capable of embracing it more.

As adults, we do laugh, just not enough.

The benefits of laughter in regulating your nervous system are really conducive to a good night's sleep. Can you recall a recent time you had with lots of laughter? How did you sleep that night?

It is not a connection we often make and yet the therapeutic value of laughter cannot be overestimated. One of my favourite sounds when I am running a retreat is the sound of laughter coming from the group. With each day, the group bonds, and the laughter gets louder.

Frequent deep belly laughs don't just feel good, they can help you live longer. A Norwegian study over a 15-year period examined the link between having a sense of humour and mortality rates among 53,556 women and men. Interestingly, the women showed an overall 48 per cent lower risk of death from all causes, a 73 per cent lower risk of dying from heart disease and 83 per cent from an infection. In men the findings showed no change apart from the risk of death by infection; it appears that the gender variation could be due to a decline in men's humour as they age.[86]

In order to laugh more, we need to connect more.

The sixth pillar in lifestyle medicine is connection and relationships. The more connected you feel to your loved ones, the safer you feel – and as you know, the safer you feel, the better you sleep.

If you have ever had a disagreement or fallen out with someone just before bed, you will know how difficult it is to get to sleep. The rush of cortisol that is created in conflict is damaging on many levels. A phrase your grandmother may have said, 'Don't let the sun go down on an argument,' is scientifically accurate. Going to bed on an argument not only makes sleep less likely to come but, fascinatingly, there is research to show that if you are angry when you go to sleep, your negative feelings will harden into resentment.[87] Negative emotional memories are harder to reverse after a night's sleep. Yunzhe Liu, who led this research at Beijing Normal University, says, 'We would suggest to first resolve the argument before going to bed; don't sleep on your anger.' On another note, the findings have also shown that going to sleep soon after a traumatic event could be linked to higher rates of post-traumatic stress disorder (PTSD). If you suffer a traumatic event, it could be worth staying up to prevent the event being reinforced in your mind.

If you do feel frustrated with a loved one, make sure to resolve the tension earlier in the day and never bring up a topic that is likely to result in a dispute before bed. One way to avoid conflict arising in the first place is to ensure that you are prioritising your relationships, from your closest connections to your more casual acquaintances. To feel that you belong is crucial to surrendering to sleep. Your relationships will naturally improve as your sleep does.

In a busy life with many responsibilities, often the most important aspects of your life, such as self-care and time with friends and family, come way down on your list. This is so common and understandable, yet many of us pay the price of having a lack of connection in our lives. The price is a lack of laughter.

From a biological perspective, when you are lonely you fall out of homeostasis (a steady, balanced internal, physical, chemical and social state). Isolation, whether it is genuine or perceived, creates a craving to be with other people and this causes the body to go into a stress response. When we spend too much time disconnected from our fellow human beings, the molecule tachykinin builds up, and this can cause us to become socially awkward and even hostile or paranoid.

A very unfortunate cycle commences: the longer we spend isolated, the more difficult we find it to connect. John Cacioppo, a social neuroscientist specialising in the impact of loneliness on the brain, says that loneliness is contagious, affects one in four people and increases the chances of early death by 20 per cent.[88]

It is worth noting that social isolation and loneliness are not the same thing. You can feel lonely while attending a big social gathering; often, it is this type of loneliness that people find the hardest. Loneliness is about feeling disconnected from others and is not linked to the amount of time you spend with others. Cacioppo says fewer connections are better. The classic case is the billionaire who sees that everyone wants to be their friend, but in the billionaire's eyes, there is doubt: are their relationships genuine or are they motivated by material gain?

The impact of Covid-19 and the multiple lockdowns, where most people across the world experienced increased levels of loneliness, has yet to be fully seen. A Welsh public health study looking at 8,960 adults from a cross-section of the population showed significant regression in self-reported feelings of loneliness, along with a decline in physical and mental health compared to pre-pandemic feelings. The findings showed that women under 35 years of age were most at risk of loneliness, as well as those with chronic health conditions.[89]

For teenagers and children at key developmental stages in their social development, it is too soon to say what the long-term impacts of the Covid-19 lockdowns are. However, I have seen many young people present in my clinic with confidence and self-esteem issues since the pandemic. If you have children whom you think may have been affected, it is important to keep a close eye on them and seek professional help if necessary.

The most essential way to connect meaningfully with others is to spend time connecting to and with yourself. If you are a person who loves your own company, great, but make sure that you also spend time with people who uplift and care for you. If you find it hard to be on your own and crave a lot of social interaction, challenge yourself to spend time alone. Extrovert or introvert, it is all about balance. It is not about the number of friendships you have, but it is about the quality. Laughter, like sleep, needs to come organically, so make sure to seek out those people who are naturally prone to finding humour in life.

What this Looks Like for Me

They say that if you love what you do, you never work a day in your life. I agree with this; however, connection and finding time for the people I love is always the lifestyle pillar that needs my attention. I can become consumed with my work as it matters a lot to me. I do always bring humour to what I do, and encourage my one-to-one clients and groups to embrace laughter. I am an extrovert who loves to spend time alone. There was a time when I would have done anything not to be on my own, but now I crave it. When I retreat into myself, I always come out better and more in a position to laugh with anyone who is willing to join in!

Reflective Journaling Prompts

✦ When do you feel most at peace? Describe in detail the circumstances, and the place. Are you alone or with people?

✦ When was a time that you practised non-attachment to a possession? When did you practise non-attachment to an outcome?

✦ How do you want to feel at the end of your life? What would prevent you from cultivating this now?

✦ ✦ ✦

Positive Practice

HOLD YOURSELF ACCOUNTABLE with compassion for any secondary gains you may have from being 'a bad sleeper' or not prioritising your sleep. Remember to bring self-compassion to anything you notice.

✦ ✦ ✦

Affirmations to Repeat

✦ 'I have enough. I am enough.'

✦ 'Inner peace is within me.'

✦ 'I rest in peace each night.'

✦ 'I wake in joy each morning.'

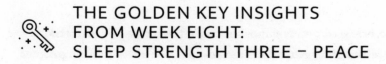

THE GOLDEN KEY INSIGHTS FROM WEEK EIGHT: SLEEP STRENGTH THREE – PEACE

✦ Peace is contentment. No striving or yearning for more is necessary. This moment is enough, you have enough, your life is enough, and you are enough.

- Resistance to being fully satisfied in your life is part of being human, it is not your fault and it is part of the primitive survival brain that is designed to seek more. To help you with this, remember that contentment is not complacency; inner peace is the springboard for continued success and happiness.

- Practising non-attachment not only to your possessions but also to the external outcomes in your life ensures that peace is always present. This takes a lot of mindful practice. Please note each time you are able to do this, for example when you are waiting for the sale of a house to complete and need to detach from whether it goes ahead or not. You continue to live in peace.

- Donald Winnicott's 'false self' is born in childhood when a child does not feel accepted for who they are but rather as a construct that suits the parent. Are you aware of your conditioned self? It is time to accept and love yourself just as you are – this brings peace, not arrogance.

- Amid the busyness of your external life there is serenity. The deeper you sleep, the more you can access peace in your waking hours and stay calm even when things are chaotic.

- Please ensure you have listened to the night-time audios for eight weeks. Remember that they are available to you as a life-time tool.

So, here we are at the end of Week Eight. How do you feel? In the conclusion, I will share how you can continue your Sleep Well journey. The audios that you have been listening to you are available as a lifetime tool. You can return to the start of the programme at any stage, especially if you enter a new life challenge that causes your sleep and life to go out of balance. Remember, I am always here if you find that you need extra guidance.

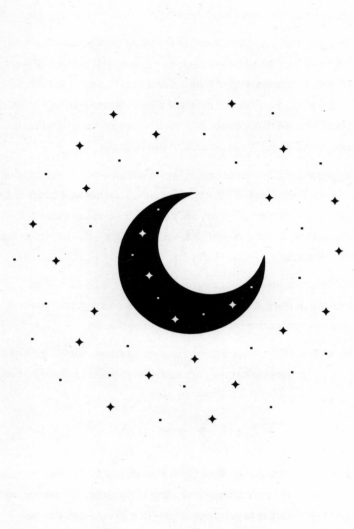

SHARING YOUR LIGHT

If the Sun and Moon should ever doubt, they'd immediately go out.

WILLIAM BLAKE

✦ ✦ ✦

Measure Your Sleep

PLEASE TAKE A moment to give your final sleep rating.

On a scale of 0 to 10, how well have you slept in the last week? (0 is 'terribly' and 10 is 'very well'.) Please use the image below to mark where you feel you are on this scale.

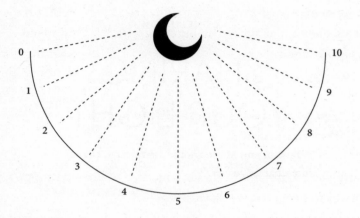

Please take a moment to compare this number with the very first measurement you took on page 7.

Returning to Your Best-Slept Self

I WROTE THIS book to help you to wake up to the beauty of your life, which can only be seen in its full magnificence through well-slept eyes. Bring to mind the image of yourself in the mirror that you first visualised in Week One. Your beautiful self, full of positive energy. If you have engaged with the programme, this image is no longer a projection into the future, a distant dream or a figment of your imagination. It has become a present reality. You are glowing, vibrant, and bursting with life. You spend your days awake and your nights asleep, just as nature always intended for you.

> **You have awakened to the life of peace and joy that you deserve.**

Thank you so much for allowing me to guide you through the doorway to sleep. You now have the golden key. This key can never be lost now that your relationship with sleep has been transformed into one that is built on mutual respect and love. You will continue to benefit from this relationship as long as you live. It will heal you; it will pick you up each time you fall, and it will keep on giving you an abundance of health and happiness. You know that all you need to do is let go, surrender and trust sleep to do what it does best – give you life.

As you continue to sleep well, your emotions have become more balanced and life's multitude of minor irritations no longer disturb you in the same way. You now place your precious attention on rest, relaxation and sleeping peacefully. As you have discovered, this is a book about self-compassion and being present, patient and peaceful so that you can sleep well.

You are present, patient and at peace.

There was an indie movie many years ago called *The Book That Wrote Itself*. How I wish this were true! However, a book does in one sense give birth to itself. It evolves through the writing process and the author is often a conduit for a message that needs to be heard. This doesn't mean the writer is not engaged in the process; like a child, a book requires immense devotion and energy to bring it to fruition. Researching sleep science has required immense presence and patience. Ultimately, it has led me to a peace that is very profound.

As I wrote the book, my sleep transformed – we have come on this journey together.

I've woken up to the true value of sleep. I can see the difference between 'OK sleep' and 'magnificent sleep'. I feel the abundance of energy and life that consistent deep sleep brings. I refuse to revert to taking sleep for granted when it is 'good' and then being frustrated when it is 'bad'. Sleep deserves better than that, and so do you. I know that for my sleep to continue to function so well, I need to love and cherish it. I know that to continue to awaken, I need to continue to sleep serenely.

I have utter confidence in the eight sleep habits and principles of this book. I know that the Sleep Well Formula (Breathe + Imagine + Experience = Faith) works because I have used it with many clients and I practise it every night, even though, for the most part, I am no longer aware I am doing this. I know these things; what matters is that you do too.

I asked you in Week One if you have a person in your life with whom you feel safe. Someone whose breath of kindness soothes you to sleep. What did you say? When we are children and adolescents, it is the job of our parents or guardians to provide this sense of deep security, and as we slowly mature into adulthood, it becomes ours. If a loved one once comforted you to sleep, you now recreate this same warmth within. Inner peace allows you to let go, to die to the day and start afresh in the morning, to operate in Tolle's clock time, and live in the eternal now. You are free to be more than you do, to refrain from throwing extra arrows at yourself, to cry when you need to, to laugh often and to take the very best care of yourself that you can.

> **What a privilege it is to be given a fresh start
> every 24 hours.**

Always remember that sleep, like anything in life, is not perfect. It is as good as it can be given your current circumstances, sometimes sublime and sometimes sufficient. The quality of your sleep relies on your consistent care. You now have a wealth of scientific tools and strategies, not to mention your night-time audios, that will continue to support you. These techniques and audios become less necessary over time; sleep is, after all, innate.

Even something that is innate, like your breath, still needs your attention to function at its best. If you experience consistent good sleep, it can become easy to take it for granted, until you are met with a challenge. If your sleep becomes disrupted for any reason, if you suffer the loss of a person you love or your health, if you experience acute or chronic stress, be patient with yourself and your sleep. Reinforce the eight Sleep Well habits; they will see you through the pain and back into the light. It is also possible to begin the programme again at any stage if you feel you need the extra guidance or a refresher on the habits. The Sleep Well Programme is always there to serve as a friendly reminder of what you already know. Faith is unshakable, but habits can be broken when our life changes, so please don't hesitate to come back and visit any time.

✦ ✦ ✦

Optimise Your Sleep Experience

HERE ARE A few more final sleep suggestions to help you maximise your sleep and to build on your continued journey of sleeping well.

GO TO BED WHEN YOU ARE SLEEPY, NOT FATIGUED

Know the difference between sleepiness and fatigue. Sleepiness or drowsiness is the extreme desire to fall asleep. Sleepiness builds the longer you are awake. When you are in a routine, you will feel sleepy at the same time (more or less) each night. Sleepiness is connected to your 'sleep drive': this is the build-up of a chemical in the brain called adenosine.[90] When adenosine reaches its peak, you will have an overwhelming desire for sleep right before the onset of drifting off. Signals of this are yawning, watering eyes and difficulty keeping your eyes open.

Fatigue, on the other hand, is when you are mentally and/ or physically drained but not ready to sleep. Your brain is still wired up and often when you try to sleep it will take longer. If you experience regular fatigue, it means that your sleep is not restoring you. Habit Two 'Create a "Blissful Hour" 60-Minute

Bedtime Routine' is designed to gradually move you from fatigue to sleepiness.

QUESTION YOUR ANXIETY BEFORE A BIG EVENT

If you have a big event the next day or an early start due to travel, write out any negative or stressful thoughts you have that could cause disruption to your sleep.

For example, you might be thinking, 'I will miss the flight if I sleep in.' Question this rationally: how likely is this if you have set a clock and have a backup? Trust that you have everything organised. Another example is 'I will mess up the presentation tomorrow if I am too anxious.' Again ask yourself, is this true? Recall the last time you spoke in public and how it turned out a lot better than you thought it would. Even positive events, such as a wedding or a celebration, can cause short-term stress, so again, question how rational your concerns are.

DON'T BE A NEWS JUNKIE

Getting sucked into arresting headlines that are designed to grab your attention (known in the media as 'clickbait') will not help you to sleep peacefully. Stay informed on your terms and don't consume news or social media unconsciously. Make sure you have all notifications turned off on your phone and unfollow any people or media who elicit a feeling of unease or anxiety in your mind. Make sure the news on the radio is not constantly on in the background as this can lead to you absorbing it without intending to. Choose to stay informed (if you wish) by selecting podcasts and articles that are unbiased and give a wider perspective of what is going on in the world. The news is predominantly negative and this paints a black and unrealistic view of the world and humanity. Also, avoid watching violent or depressing dramas and films, especially before bed.

Overall, be very selective about the information you consume. In the same way you choose what to eat, choose to ingest as much positive and uplifting content as you can.

ADAPT BEFORE YOU CHANGE TIME ZONES

If you are travelling to a different time zone, gradually shift your sleeping and waking times closer to those of your new destination. This will help your body adapt more easily to the new schedule when you arrive, even if the time difference is just two hours. For example, when I go to Greece (which is two hours ahead), I start to go to bed later before I leave. Drink plenty of water before and during your flight and avoid caffeine and alcohol. Also adjust your mealtimes before you go, to get closer to the new time zone.

As soon as you arrive and it is practicable, take your shoes off and stand on the earth. This will root you in the new country. Then begin to rise, sleep and eat in the time zone that you are in. Even tweaking your routines slightly before you go will help minimise jet lag.

DON'T OVERSLEEP

Sleeping too much, also known as hypersomnia, is usually caused by a lack of effective and/or sufficient sleep. Don't try to compensate for a late night by oversleeping, as this will throw you off your rhythm and it will take you longer to get back into your regular pattern.[91] More than nine hours for a healthy adult is seen as too much. Keep in mind, healthy teenagers can need to sleep regularly for up to ten hours.[92] If you do regularly sleep more than nine hours and find that you are not refreshed, it is really worth speaking to your doctor, as it could be a sign of an underlying health condition and/or depression.

AVOID OBSESSING OVER YOUR SLEEP

There is a fine line between love and obsession. When we care for children, this line needs to be clear. Obsessing over every little issue the child may have, fussing over the details, is not beneficial – it is over-protective. This level of intense care can create the very opposite result we intend, namely an anxious child. What is true for a child also applies to your subconscious mind and hence your sleep.

Always bring your three sleep strengths to the fore: presence, patience and peace. Many people get obsessive about sleep, insisting that certain criteria MUST be met for them to sleep. While the eight habits in the programme are designed to create the optimum circumstances for sleep, there will be times when you can't do some or any of them. You may be required to share a room at an event, to fly through the night with a baby crying in the seat right behind you, be exposed to a wedding party in the hotel you booked for peace and quiet, have a teenager who is out late and hasn't called, or be needed to care for a loved one. It is at these times that a flexible approach is needed. When you accept the challenge (if there is nothing you can do to improve it), your sleep may not be as high in quality as usual; it will, however, be better than you may have imagined. When your routine is disrupted the most important thing to hold on to is your faith. Your faith is unshakable in the face of any changes and inconsistency. Trust it.

CREATE A SLEEP-AID PACK

A sleep-aid pack can really deepen your sleep. In my sleep-aid pack, I have my eye mask, earplugs and my teddy! I know, don't laugh – but the softness and smell of my teddy help to induce a feeling of comfort. The eye mask keeps the room beautifully dark and is very helpful when it gets light at 5 a.m.! The earplugs have probably, on occasion, saved my marriage. It is important not to become attached to these items (this is also the case for your night-time audio). If you find yourself without one or more of them, your faith in your ability to sleep remains the same.

SLOW DOWN YOUR MIND FIRST THING IN THE MORNING

As soon as you rise, start to slow the thoughts in your mind. When you do this, you start the day as you intend to go on, in presence, rather than being consumed by thought. This early intervention will help you bring focus and clarity to your day and set the stage for letting go at night. Your 'Start Your Day in Stillness' morning meditation is designed to help you with this.

TAKE A MAGNESIUM SUPPLEMENT BEFORE BED

Please note that you should always consult a doctor before taking any supplement. There are many potential benefits of taking a magnesium supplement 30–60 minutes before you go to sleep, as it can deepen the quality of your sleep.[93] I find this to be the case. Magnesium acts as a muscle relaxant and can help people who suffer from restless leg syndrome.[94] Magnesium also helps regulate GABA (a neurotransmitter that promotes relaxation and sleep) receptors, enhancing the effects of GABA in the brain and promoting a sense of calmness. Adequate levels of magnesium can support the natural production of melatonin, helping to synchronise the body's internal clock and promote a regular sleep schedule.

PRACTISE AFFIRMATIONS

Create your own, use some of the ones suggested already in Presence, Patience and Peace, or take your pick from below. Please note some of these have been interspersed through your audios and will be familiar to you already on a subconscious level.

I recommend consciously choosing to write three down per night and using the same ones until they become automatic. As you write them, it is essential to feel them in your body. If some of them don't feel totally true to you, select the ones that resonate with you most.

+ 'I am full of love as I drift to sleep.'

+ 'I am letting go of this day with an open and joyous heart.'

+ 'As I sleep, I dream, and as I dream, I find my true self.'

+ 'I am awakening to the reality of who I am: pure love.'

+ 'I radiate compassion for everyone I encounter.'

+ 'I am a vessel of love, compassion and forgiveness, spreading positivity wherever I go.'

+ 'I am at peace with all that has passed and all that will come.'

+ 'My source of joy is within me.'

+ 'My source of joy is in my smile.'

+ 'As I sleep, I make sense of the world and find the guidance I seek.'

+ 'I am grateful for the abundance of blessings in my life, both seen and unseen.'

- ✦ 'I am connected to a higher power that guides and supports me in all aspects of my life.'

- ✦ 'I trust that the universe is unfolding exactly as it should, and I am a part of its divine plan.'

- ✦ 'I am deserving of love and happiness, and I allow them to flow abundantly into my life.'

- ✦ 'When I rise, I will bring the whole universe with me.'

- ✦ 'I am at one with myself, others and the world.'

- ✦ 'My life is a blessing and I value it with love and respect.'

- ✦ 'I choose to sleep peacefully so I can shine brightly.'

- ✦ 'I greet tomorrow with a smile, knowing that my positive energy will touch the lives of others.'

- ✦ 'Each day is a fresh start for happiness, and tomorrow I choose to create a beautiful and fulfilling day.'

✦ ✦ ✦

Share Your Light

Don't you know yet, it is your light that lights the world?

RUMI

AS I WRITE these final words, I am blessed to be in my spiritual home, Greece. The light here is startlingly luminous; I have yet to visit another country where the light is quite so bright. It brings everything and everyone to life.

Can you see this light is also within you?

The story *Jonathan Livingston Seagull* by Richard Bach tells the story of an ambitious and adventurous seagull whose main aim in life is to do something worthwhile, to soar above his conditioning. He is determined to rise above the expectations his family and flock have for him, and practises flying higher than any other seagull, soon learning to reach the utmost heights of the blue sky. Livingston is far from praised for his success and is ostracised by his community. He remains undeterred and flies even higher to meet more like-minded seagulls who have gone before him. Rather than abandon his roots, Livingston returns to them and begins a training academy that teaches the courageous among them how to fly just as high.

Now that you are well-slept, your light, your magnificence, has the potential to shine through. Please share the Sleep Well Programme with everyone you can. As you do this you may meet rebuttals from others who have resigned themselves to a life half-slept. This resignation is an acceptance that leads to a full stop rather than a new beginning. Your voice may be the one that opens the door to change.

Inspire others with your presence, patience and peace.

You now belong to a new tribe of well-slept awakened people who have the power to elevate the collective consciousness, activate positive change and make the world lighter. Sleep now, like you live and breathe, with gratitude and grace. No doubt. No questions. Just faith.

ACKNOWLEDGEMENTS

Thank you, Ciaran and Luca. Your presence and patience give me so much peace. It cannot be easy to live with someone who is writing a book, especially one on sleep! Your good humour, encouragement and endless chats allowed me to keep going. Your continued support allows me to help others and your love keeps me strong.

Thank you to my clients who have taught me so much about what it means to be human. Without you, there would be no book. Really, I owe so much to each and every one of you.

Thanks to my mum, dad and sister Orla, some of the best sleepers I know! Thanks for sending me lots of *Guardian* articles on the latest sleep science; your support is always so evident and appreciated.

Thank you to my friend and fellow wellness leader Dermot Whelan for writing the foreword to this book. You are always so generous with your time. I have watched in awe as you have transformed your own life and thousands of others with mindful devotion and love.

To my faithful friend Jane McDaid for teaching me what it means to be a really good sleeper. All your suggestions over the years must have finally sunk in and I felt compelled to write this book. We now speak the same 'sleep language' and I understand the 'secret' to your abundant health and energy.

Thank you to the incredible team at Gill and in particular my editor, Sarah Liddy, for believing in me when I wrote my first book, *The Positive Habit*, five years ago. It was a big step for me and I am overjoyed at the success it has had in helping people. Thanks to Aoibheann Molumby for being a remarkable book midwife. Your tenacity and skill are second to none and I am so grateful for your editing skills. Both yourself and Sarah have brought this book to where it needs to be. Thanks to Charlie Lawlor and Graham Thew for your excellent design work. Thanks to the marketing team and publicist Fiona Murphy for doing the incredibly vital job of getting the book 'out there'. Thanks for a thorough copy-edit by Esther Ní Dhonnacha.

Thanks so much to Fionnuala Sherry, who generously shared her story so that she could help others to sleep well. Fionnuala, you are a beacon of light in the world. Never doubt it.

Thank you to Dr Sarah McKay for your extensive interview, expert help and time. You remind me of my friend Jane, and your ability to care for yourselves and others is an inspiration for us all.

Sat Bir Singh Khalsa, I am so grateful for your interview and sharing your wisdom. It meant so much to secure an interview with you. Thank you.

Thanks to my talented yoga teacher Rohan Hennessy and author of the Rest Ritual. You teach with presence, patience and peace. Your shavasana should win awards, although I do know yoga (like sleep) is not a competition. Thanks also to my community in YogaHub and in particular Sile Nolan for supporting my books.

Thanks to my Keep The Light retreat group. The sense of love and community you create lifts my heart each day.

Thanks to Karen Kelly for the best massages in the world; your healing hands helped me cope with too much time on the computer.

Thanks also to my close group of friends for listening to me as I spoke about the book and no doubt drove them slowly mad. Your support and laughter always lift me up.

Finally, I thank both myself for writing this book and, most important, YOU the reader for your faith. Together we are powerful beyond measure.

NOTES

1   The average rate of heritability of insomnia is 37 per cent; however, this does not mean that expression of those genes is activated. Your lifestyle and mindset are key to keeping them dormant.

2   American College of Lifestyle Medicine (2023). Available: https://lifestylemedicine.org/.

3   Kris-Etherton, P. M., Eckel, R. H., Howard, B. V., St Jeor, S., & Bazzarre, T. L. (2001). Lyon Diet Heart Study. *Circulation*, *103*(13), 1823–1825. https://doi.org/10.1161/01.cir.103.13.1823

4   Hari, J. (2022). Your attention didn't collapse. It was stolen. *The Guardian*, March 8. https://www.theguardian.com/science/2022/jan/02/attention-span-focus-screens-apps-smartphones-social-media

5   Deloitte (2017). Smartphones are useful but they can be distracting. https://www2.deloitte.com/content/dam/Deloitte/global/Images/infographics/technologymediatelecommunications/gx-deloitte-tmt-2018-smartphones-report.pdf

6   Lupton, D., & Jutel, A. (2015). Self-tracking, social media and personal health management: a qualitative study. *Journal of Health Psychology*, 20(7), 1154–1163.

7   Dr. Gina Poe: Use Sleep to Enhance Learning, Memory & Emotional State – Huberman Lab. (2023, December 6). https://www.hubermanlab.com/episode/dr-gina-poe-use-sleep-to-enhance-learning-memory-and-emotional-state

8   McGill University (n.d.). The Brain from Top to Bottom. https://thebrain.mcgill.ca/flash/d/d_11/d_11_cr/d_11_cr_cyc/d_11_cr_cyc.html

9   Tseng, Y., Zhao, B., Liu, J., Ding, H., Wang, F., & Wang, L. (2020). Sleep deprivation and adrenalectomy lead to enhanced innate escape response to visual looming stimuli. *Biochemical and Biophysical Research Communications*, *527*(3), 737–743. https://doi.org/10.1016/j.bbrc.2020.04.061

10   Huffington, A. S. (2016). *The Sleep Revolution: transforming your life, one night at a time.* https://openlibrary.org/books/OL27203004M/The_sleep_revolution

11   Gavriloff, D., Sheaves, B., Juss, A., Espie, C. A., Miller, C. H., & Kyle, S. D. (2018). Sham sleep feedback delivered via actigraphy biases daytime symptom reports in people with insomnia: Implications for insomnia disorder and wearable devices. *Journal of Sleep Research*, *27*(6). https://doi.org/10.1111/jsr.12726

12   'Demystifying The Female Brain With Dr Sarah McKay', Interview with Dr Ben Webber, 2020. https://www.youtube.com/watch?v=zW3uJIAdyHE

13   *MSUToday* (2017, September 14). 'For worriers, expressive writing cools brain on stressful tasks'. *MSUToday*, Michigan State University. https://msutoday.msu.edu/news/2017/for-worriers-expressive-writing-cools-brain-on-stressful-tasks

14   Emmons, R.A. and McCullough, M.E. (2003). Counting blessings versus burdens: An experimental investigation of gratitude and subjective well-being in daily life. *Journal of Personality and Social Psychology*, *84*(2), 377–389. https://doi.org/10.1037/0022-3514.84.2.377.

15   Smallwood, J., & Schooler, J. W. (2015). The science of mind wandering: Empirically navigating the stream of consciousness. *Annual Review of Psychology*, *66*(1), 487–518. https://doi.org/10.1146/annurev-psych-010814-015331

16   Balban, M. Y., Neri, E., Kogon, M., Weed, L., Nouriani, B., Jo, B., Holl, G., Zeitzer, J. M., Spiegel, D., & Huberman, A. D. (2023). Brief structured respiration practices enhance mood and reduce physiological arousal. *Cell Reports Medicine*, *4*(1), 100895. https://doi.org/10.1016/j.xcrm.2022.100895

17   Gloster, A. T., Walder, N., Levin, M. E., Twohig, M. P., & Karekla, M. (2020). The empirical status of acceptance and commitment therapy: A review of meta-analyses. *Journal of Contextual Behavioral Science*, *18*, 181–192. https://doi.org/10.1016/j.jcbs.2020.09.009

18   Gračanin, A., Bylsma, L. M., & Vingerhoets, A. (2014). Is crying a self-soothing behavior? *Frontiers in Psychology*, *5*. https://doi.org/10.3389/fpsyg.2014.00502

19   Millings, A., Hepper, E. G., Hart, C. M., Swift, L., & Rowe, A. C. (2016). Holding back the tears: Individual differences in adult crying proneness reflect attachment orientation and attitudes to crying. *Frontiers in Psychology*, *7*. https://doi.org/10.3389/fpsyg.2016.01003

20   Sung, K., Khan, S., Nawaz, M. S., Cerniglia, C. E., Tamplin, M. L., Phillips, R. W., & Kelley, L. C. (2011). Lysozyme as a barrier to growth of *Bacillus anthracis* strain Sterne in liquid egg white, milk and beef. *Food Microbiology*, *28*(6), 1231–1234. https://doi.org/10.1016/j.fm.2011.03.002

21   Chatterjee, R. (2023, June 1). *How Your Brain Creates Your Reality: A Neuroscientist's Take On Consciousness, Near Death Experiences & What it Really Means to be You with Professor Anil Seth.* https://drchatterjee.com/how-your-brain-creates-your-reality-a-neuroscientists-take-on-consciousness-near-death-experiences-what-it-really-means-to-be-you-with-professor-anil-seth/

22   https://pubmed.ncbi.nlm.nih.gov/?term=sleep&filter=years.1981-2023

23   Hill, T. D., DeAngelis, R. T., & Ellison, C. G. (2018). Religious involvement as a social determinant of sleep: An initial review and conceptual model. *Sleep Health*, *4*(4), 325–330. https://doi.org/10.1016/j.sleh.2018.04.001

24   World Health Organization (2022). *Global Status Report on Physical Activity 2022.* https://www.who.int/teams/health-promotion/physical-activity/global-status-report-on-physical-activity-2022

25   Gonzalez, J. T., Veasey, R. C., Rumbold, P. L. S., & Stevenson, E. (2013). Breakfast and exercise contingently affect postprandial metabolism and energy balance in physically active males. *British Journal of Nutrition*, *110*(4), 721–732. https://doi.org/10.1017/s0007114512005582

26   Nobari, H., Azarian, S., Saedmocheshi, S., et al. (2023) Narrative review: The role of circadian rhythm on sports performance, hormonal regulation, immune system function, and injury prevention in athletes. Heliyon 9(9). https://www.cell.com/heliyon/fulltext/ S2405-8440(23)06844-5. doi:10.1016/j.heliyon.2023.e19636

27   Harvard Health. (2019, April 1). Does exercising at night affect sleep? https://www.health.harvard.edu/ staying-healthy/does-exercising-at-night-affect-sleep

28   Oken, B. S. et al. (2006, February 1). *Randomized, controlled, six-month trial of yoga in healthy seniors: effects on cognition and quality of life. Alternative Therapies in Health and Medicine*, 12(1), 40–7. https://pubmed.ncbi. nlm.nih.gov/16454146/

29   Papp, M. E., Nygren-Bonnier, M., Gullstrand, L., Wändell, P., & Lindfors, P. (2019). A randomized controlled pilot study of the effects of 6-week high intensity hatha yoga protocol on health-related outcomes among students. *Journal of Bodywork and Movement Therapies*, 23(4), 766–772. https://doi. org/10.1016/j.jbmt.2019.05.013

30   NeuroHealth Associates. (2019, December 2). *The Science of Brainwaves – The Language of the Brain | NeuroHealth Associates*. https://nhahealth.com/ brainwaves-the-language

31   Ackerman, S. (1992). *The Development and Shaping of the Brain*. Discovering the Brain – NCBI Bookshelf. https://www.ncbi.nlm.nih.gov/books/NBK234146/

32   Sample, I. (2017, November 28). Sleep 'resets' brain connections crucial for memory and learning, study reveals. *The Guardian*. https://www.theguardian.com/ science/2016/aug/23/sleep-resets-brain-connections-crucial-for-memory-and-learning-study-reveals

33   Sierra-Siegert, M., Jay, E., Florez, C., & Garcia, A. E. (2016). Minding the dreamer within: An experimental study on the effects of enhanced dream recall on creative thinking. *Journal of Creative Behavior*, 53(1), 83–96. https://doi.org/10.1002/jocb.168

34   Wilbanks, J. (2023, September 15). *Nightmares – Sleep Education by American Academy of Sleep Medicine*. Sleep Education. https://sleepeducation.org/sleep-disorders/nightmares/#

35   Saunders, D., Roe, C. A., Smith, G. D., & Clegg, H. (2016). Lucid dreaming incidence: A quality effects meta-analysis of 50 years of research. *Consciousness and Cognition*, 43, 197–215. https://doi.org/10.1016/j. concog.2016.06.002

36   Baird, B., Erlacher, D., Czisch, M., Spoormaker, V. I., & Dresler, M. (2019). Consciousness and Meta-Consciousness during sleep. In *Handbook of Behavioral Neuroscience* (pp. 283–295). https://doi.org/10.1016/ b978-0-12-813743-7.00019-0

37   Brylowski, A., Levitan, L., & LaBerge, S. (1989). H-reflex suppression and autonomic activation during lucid REM sleep: A case study. *Sleep*, 12(4), 374–378. https://doi.org/10.1093/sleep/12.4.374

38   Aspy, D. J., Delfabbro, P., Proeve, M., & Mohr, P. (2017). Reality testing and the mnemonic induction of lucid dreams: Findings from the national Australian lucid dream induction study. *Dreaming*, 27(3), 206–231. https://doi.org/10.1037/drm0000059

39   O'Callaghan, F. V., Muurlink, O., and Reid, N. (2018). Effects of caffeine on sleep quality and daytime functioning. *Risk Management and Healthcare Policy*, Volume 11, 263–271. https://doi.org/10.2147/ rmhp.s156404.

40   Pacheco, D., & Pacheco, D. (2023, November 8). *Alcohol and Sleep*. Sleep Foundation. https:// www.sleepfoundation.org/nutrition/alcohol-and-sleep#references-81435

41   Stein, M. D., & Friedmann, P. D. (2006). Disturbed sleep and its relationship to alcohol use. *Substance Abuse*, 26(1), 1–13. https://doi.org/10.1300/ j465v26n01_01

42   American Academy of Sleep Medicine (2014). *The International Classification of Sleep Disorders – Third Edition* (ICSD-3). Darien, IL.

43   Matheson, E., & Hainer, B. L. (2017, July 1). *Insomnia: Pharmacologic therapy*. AAFP. https:// www.aafp.org/pubs/afp/issues/2017/0701/p29. html#afp20170701p029-b2

44   Gehrman, P., Pfeiffenberger, C., & Byrne, E. M. (2013). The role of genes in the insomnia phenotype. *Sleep Medicine Clinics*, 8(3), 323–331. https://doi.org/ 10.1016/j.jsmc.2013.04.005

45   Galavíz, K. I., Narayan, K. V., Lobelo, F., & Weber, M. B. (2015). Lifestyle and the prevention of type 2 diabetes: A status report. *American Journal of Lifestyle Medicine*, 12(1), 4–20. https://doi. org/10.1177/1559827615619159

46   Matheson, J. K. (2003c). Disorders of sleep. In *Elsevier eBooks* (pp. 962–975). https://doi.org/10.1016/ b0-44-306557-8/50152-0

47   Kawai, K., Iwamoto, K., Miyata, S., Okada, I., Ando, M., Fujishiro, H., Noda, A., & Ozaki, N. (2022). A study of factors causing sleep state misperception in patients with depression. *Nature and Science of Sleep*, Volume 14, 1273–1283. https://doi.org/10.2147/ nss.s366774

48   Jahrami, H., BaHammam, A. S., Bragazzi, N. L., Saif, Z., Faris, M. E., & Vitiello, M. V. (2021). Sleep problems during the COVID-19 pandemic by population: A systematic review and meta-analysis. *Journal of Clinical Sleep Medicine*, 17(2), 299–313. https://doi.org/10.5664/jcsm.8930

49   IARC Working Group on the Identification of Carcinogenic Hazards to Humans (2020). *Night Shift Work*. Lyon: International Agency for Research on Cancer. (IARC Monographs on the Identification of Carcinogenic Hazards to Humans, No. 124: 1. Exposure Data. https://www.ncbi.nlm.nih.gov/books/ NBK568199/

50   Blase, K., & Van Waning, A. (2019). Heart rate variability, cortisol and attention focus during Shamatha Quiescence meditation. *Applied Psychophysiology and Biofeedback*, 44(4), 331–342. https://doi.org/10.1007/s10484-019-09448-w

51   Mallampalli, M. P., & Carter, C. L. (2014). Exploring sex and gender differences in sleep health: A Society for Women's Health research report. *Journal of Womens Health*, 23(7), 553–562. https://doi. org/10.1089/jwh.2014.4816

52   Pengo, M. F., Won, C., & Bourjeily, G. (2018). Sleep in women across the life span. *Chest, 154*(1), 196–206. https://doi.org/10.1016/j.chest.2018.04.005

53   Worley, W. (2016, March 11). Women need more sleep than men because of their 'complex' brains, research suggests. *The Independent*. https://www.independent.co.uk/life-style/health-and-families/health-news/women-need-more-sleep-because-of-their-complex-brains-research-suggests-a6925266.html

54   Lee, J., Han, Y., Cho, H. H., & Kim, M. (2019). Sleep disorders and menopause. *Journal of Menopausal Medicine, 25*(2), 83. https://doi.org/10.6118/jmm.19192

55   Mayo Clinic (2023, April 6). *Sleep apnea – Symptoms and causes*. https://www.mayoclinic.org/diseases-conditions/sleep-apnea/symptoms-causes/syc-20377631

56   Central Statistics Office (CSO). (2022, September 9). *Suicide Statistics 2019*. https://www.cso.ie/en/releasesandpublications/ep/p-ss/suicidestatistics2019

57   Ilić, M., & Ilić, I. (2022). Worldwide suicide mortality trends (2000–2019): A joinpoint regression analysis. *World Journal of Psychiatry, 12*(8), 1044–1060. https://doi.org/10.5498/wjp.v12.i8.1044

58   Mayo Clinic (2022, December 21). *Male depression: Understanding the issues*. https://www.mayoclinic.org/diseases-conditions/depression/in-depth/male-depression/art-20046216

59   Schlundt, M. (2022, May 24). The long-term health implications of snoring. *Sleep Cycle alarm clock*. https://www.sleepcycle.com/snoring/long-term-snoring-health-implications/

60   Ludtke, L. (2020). Sleep disruption and the 'nightmare of total illumination' in late nineteenth- and early twentieth-century dystopian fiction. *Interface Focus, 10*(3), 20190130. https://doi.org/10.1098/rsfs.2019.0130

61   Snyder, F., et al. (1964). The effects of light on human beings. *Science 144*(3619): 1042–1048.

62   Cajochen, C., Münch, M., Kobialka, S., Kräuchi, K., Steiner, R., Oelhafen, P., Orgül, S., & Wirz-Justice, A. (2005). High sensitivity of human melatonin, alertness, thermoregulation, and heart rate to short wavelength light. *Journal of Clinical Endocrinology & Metabolism, 90*(3), 1311–1316. https://doi.org/10.1210/jc.2004-0957

63   Wright, K. P., Hughes, R. J., Kronauer, R. E., Dijk, D., & Czeisler, C. A. (2001). Intrinsic near-24-h pacemaker period determines limits of circadian entrainment to a weak synchronizer in humans. *Proceedings of the National Academy of Sciences of the United States of America, 98*(24), 14027–14032. https://doi.org/10.1073/pnas.201530198

64   An, Y., & Joo, C. (2016). The U-shaped association between self-reported sleep duration and visual impairment in Korean adults: A population-based study. *Sleep Medicine, 26*, 30–36. https://doi.org/10.1016/j.sleep.2016.08.005

65   Cohen, R., Bavishi, C., & Rozanski, A. (2016). Purpose in life and its relationship to all-cause mortality and cardiovascular events. *Psychosomatic Medicine, 78*(2), 122–133. https://doi.org/10.1097/psy.0000000000000274

66   Na, H., Ekanayake, V., Padilla, V. J., & Elkins, G. (2022). Pilot study of hypnotic relaxation therapy for well-being (HRT-WB): A new intervention to enhance well-being and positive affect. *International Journal of Clinical and Experimental Hypnosis, 70*(4), 328–349. https://doi.org/10.1080/00207144.2022.2124375

67   Huberman, A. (2022, February 21). *Dr. David Spiegel: Using Hypnosis to Enhance Health & Performance | Huberman Lab Podcast #60* [Video]. YouTube. https://www.youtube.com/watch?v=PctD-ki8dCc

68   Wise, J. (2023). Meditation statistics 2024: Popularity, industry & market size. EarthWeb. https://earthweb.com/meditation-statistics/

69   Hepsomali, P., Groeger, J. A., Nishihira, J., & Scholey, A. (2020b). Effects of oral gamma-aminobutyric acid (GABA) administration on stress and sleep in humans: A systematic review. *Frontiers in Neuroscience, 14*. https://doi.org/10.3389/fnins.2020.00923

70   Kim, S., Jo, K., Hong, K. T., Han, S. H., & Suh, H. J. (2019). GABA and l-theanine mixture decreases sleep latency and improves NREM sleep. *Pharmaceutical Biology, 57*(1), 64–72. https://doi.org/10.1080/13880209.2018.1557698

71   Johns Hopkins Medicine (n.d.). Vital Signs (Body Temperature, Pulse Rate, Respiration Rate, Blood Pressure). https://www.hopkinsmedicine.org/health/conditions-and-diseases/vital-signs-body-temperature-pulse-rate-respiration-rate-blood-pressure

72   Russo, M., Santarelli, D. M., & O'Rourke, D. (2017). The physiological effects of slow breathing in the healthy human. *Breathe, 13*(4), 298–309. https://doi.org/10.1183/20734735.009817

73   Zaccaro, A., Piarulli, A., Laurino, M., Garbella, E., Menicucci, D., Neri, B., & Gemignani, A. (2018). How breath-control can change your life: A systematic review on psycho-physiological correlates of slow breathing. *Frontiers in Human Neuroscience, 12*. https://doi.org/10.3389/fnhum.2018.00353

74   World Health Organization (WHO). (2023, September 16). *Noncommunicable diseases*. https://www.who.int/news-room/fact-sheets/detail/noncommunicable-diseases#:~

75   Killingsworth, M. R., & Gilbert, D. T. (2010). A wandering mind is an unhappy mind. *Science, 330*(6006), 932. https://doi.org/10.1126/science.1192439

76   Schutter, N., Holwerda, T. J., Comijs, H. C., Stek, M. L., Peen, J., & Dekker, J. (2022). Loneliness, social network size and mortality in older adults: A meta-analysis. *European Journal of Ageing, 19*(4), 1057–1076. https://doi.org/10.1007/s10433-022-00740-z

77   Schnitker, S. A. (2012). An examination of patience and well-being. *Journal of Positive Psychology, 7*(4), 263–280. https://doi.org/10.1080/17439760.2012.697185

78   Mischel, W., Ebbesen, E. B., & Zeiss, A. M. (1972). Cognitive and attentional mechanisms in delay of gratification. *Journal of Personality and Social Psychology, 21*(2), 204–218. https://doi.org/10.1037/h0032198

79 Mischel, W., Shoda, Y., & Rodríguez, M. (1989). Delay of gratification in children. *Science, 244*(4907), 933–938. https://doi.org/10.1126/science.2658056

80 Blue Zones (2021, May 4). *Ikaria, Greece.* https://www.bluezones.com/explorations/ikaria-greece/

81 Naska, A., Oikonomou, E., Trichopoulou, A., Psaltopoulou, T., & Trichopoulos, D. (2007). Siesta in healthy adults and coronary mortality in the general population. *Archives of Internal Medicine, 167*(3), 296. https://doi.org/10.1001/archinte.167.3.296

82 Rönnlund, M., Åström, E., Westlin, W., Flodén, L., Unger, A., Papastamatelou, J., & Carelli, M. G. (2021). A time to sleep well and be contented: Time perspective, sleep quality, and life satisfaction. *Frontiers in Psychology, 12.* https://doi.org/10.3389/fpsyg.2021.627836

83 Lee, Y. C., Lin, Y. C., Huang, C. L., & Fredrickson, B. L. (2012). The construct and measurement of peace of mind. *Journal of Happiness Studies, 14*(2), 571–590. https://doi.org/10.1007/s10902-012-9343-5

84 Brickman, P., Coates, D., & Janoff-Bulman, R. (1978). Lottery winners and accident victims: Is happiness relative? *Journal of Personality and Social Psychology, 36*(8), 917–927. https://doi.org/10.1037/0022-3514.36.8.917

85 Neff, K. D., & Vonk, R. (2008). Self-compassion versus global self-esteem: Two different ways of relating to oneself. *Journal of Personality, 77*(1), 23–50. https://doi.org/10.1111/j.1467-6494.2008.00537.x

86 Romundstad, S., Svebak, S., Holen, A., & Holmen, J. (2016). A 15-year follow-up study of sense of humor and causes of mortality. *Psychosomatic Medicine, 78*(3), 345–353. https://doi.org/10.1097/psy.0000000000000275

87 Liu, Y., Lin, W., Liu, C., Luo, Y., Wu, J., Bayley, P. J., & Qin, S. (2016). Memory consolidation reconfigures neural pathways involved in the suppression of emotional memories. *Nature Communications, 7*(1). https://doi.org/10.1038/ncomms13375

88 Adams, T. (2019, January 25). John Cacioppo: 'Loneliness is like an iceberg – it goes deeper than we can see.' *The Guardian.* https://www.theguardian.com/science/2016/feb/28/loneliness-is-like-an-iceberg-john-cacioppo-social-neuroscience-interview

89 Allen, J., Darlington, O., Hughes, K. et al. (2022). The public health impact of loneliness during the COVID-19 pandemic. *BMC Public Health* 22, 1654 (2022). https://doi.org/10.1186/s12889-022-14055-2

90 Lazarus, M., Oishi, Y., Bjorness, T. E., & Greene, R. (2019). Gating and the need for sleep: Dissociable effects of adenosine A1 and A2A receptors. *Frontiers in Neuroscience, 13.* https://doi.org/10.3389/fnins.2019.00740

91 Johns Hopkins Medicine (2023, October 4). *Oversleeping: bad for your health?* https://www.hopkinsmedicine.org/health/wellness-and-prevention/oversleeping-bad-for-your-health#:

92 Parker, H. (2008, July 23). *Physical side effects of oversleeping.* WebMD. https://www.webmd.com/sleep-disorders/physical-side-effects-oversleeping

93 Chen, P., Bornhorst, J., Patton, S. M., Bagai, K., Nitin, R., Miah, M. R., Hare, D. J., Kysenius, K., Crouch, P. J., Xiong, L., Rouleau, G. A., Schwerdtle, T., Connor, J. R., Aschner, M., Bowman, A. B., & Walters, A. S. (2020). A potential role for zinc in restless legs syndrome. *Sleep, 44*(4). https://doi.org/10.1093/sleep/zsaa236

94 Górska, N., Słupski, J., Szałach, Ł. P., Włodarczyk, A., Szarmach, J., Jakuszkowiak-Wojten, K., Gałuszko-Węgielnik, M., Wilkowska, A., Wiglusz, M. S., & Cubała, W. J. (2019). Magnesium and ketamine in the treatment of depression. *Psychiatria Danubina, 31*(Suppl 3), 549–553.